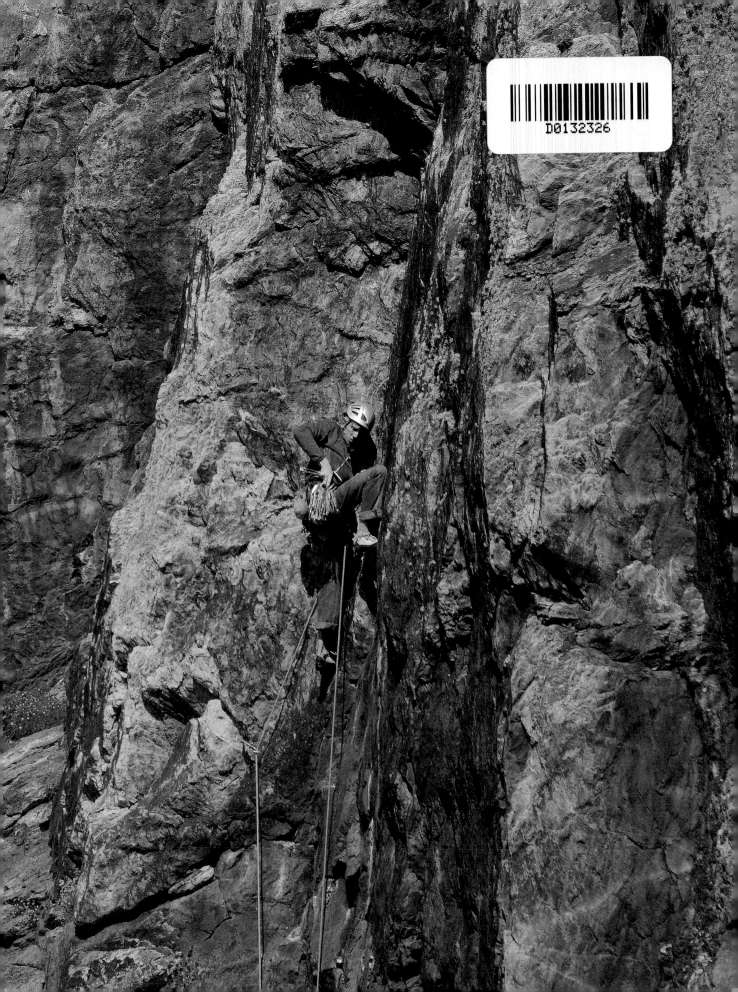

First published in April 2014

Nigel Shepherd has asserted his moral right to be identified as the author of this work.

A catalogue record for this book is available from the British Library

ISBN 978 0 85733 310 0

Library of Congress control no. 2013955822

Published by Haynes Publishing, Sparkford, Yeovil, Somerset BA22 7JJ, UK
Tel: 01963 442030 Fax: 01963 440001
Int. tel: +44 1963 442030 Int. fax: +44 1963 440001
E-mail: sales@haynes.co.uk
Website: www.haynes.co.uk

Haynes North America Inc.
861 Lawrence Drive, Newbury Park,
California 91320, USA

While every effort is taken to ensure the accuracy of the information given in this book, no liability can be accepted by the author or publishers for any loss, damage or injury caused by errors in, or omissions from the information given.

Printed in the USA by Odcombe Press LP,
1299 Bridgestone Parkway, La Vergne, TN 37086

AUTHOR'S ACKNOWLEDGEMENTS

I can't imagine how difficult it might have been to write this book without the generosity and advice offered by friends, family and colleagues. I'm deeply indebted to lots of people but would particularly like to mention a few here.

Chris Rowland (DMM), John Samways (Lyon Equipment/La Sportiva) and Dave Brown (DB Outdoor/Edelrid) very kindly gave me equipment to use in the illustrations.

Thanks to Giles Thurston for allowing me to use his table of International Grading System Comparisons, which is a carefully considered and easily interpreted piece of work on a potentially contentious subject!

Ray Wood, Dave 'Cubby' Cuthbertson, Neil Gresham and Simon Panton kindly responded to my requests for images and they all provided inspiring photos that offer a true flavour of this great sport.

Garry Smith also provided great images as well as lots of helpful advice. He spent more than a few hours of his time helping me set up and shoot some of the technical illustrations.

Libby Peter has been a sounding board for ideas and suggestions and was always keen to help with pictures and offer technical advice.

Frank Corner (my father-in-law) has a great collection of pictures from the 'old days' and kindly allowed me to use a few of them to illustrate how climbing once was. He has been climbing for seven decades and his enthusiasm remains undiminished!

Molly, Jack and Dan Shepherd, Zoe and Ruby Wood, and Lou Neill were all coerced at various stages to appear in photos – thank you all for your patience!

Any plaudits are theirs to share but I'll take full responsibility for everything else.

My thanks also to Steve and Gill at the Beacon Climbing Centre in North Wales for kindly allowing me to take photographs at the climbing wall. You have an amazing facility!

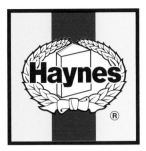

CLIMBING MANUAL

THE ESSENTIAL GUIDE TO ROCK CLIMBING

NIGEL SHEPHERD

GETTING STARTED ■ TECHNIQUES ■ KNOTS ■ SAFETY ■ PROTECTION ■ ABSEILING

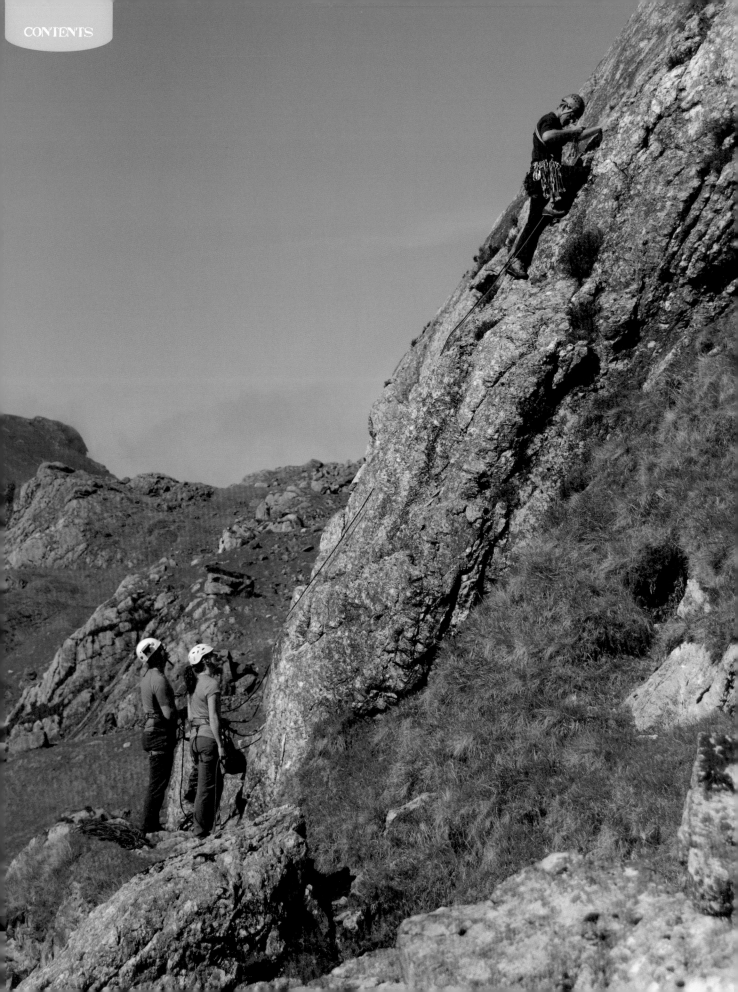

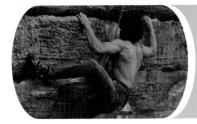

CONTENTS

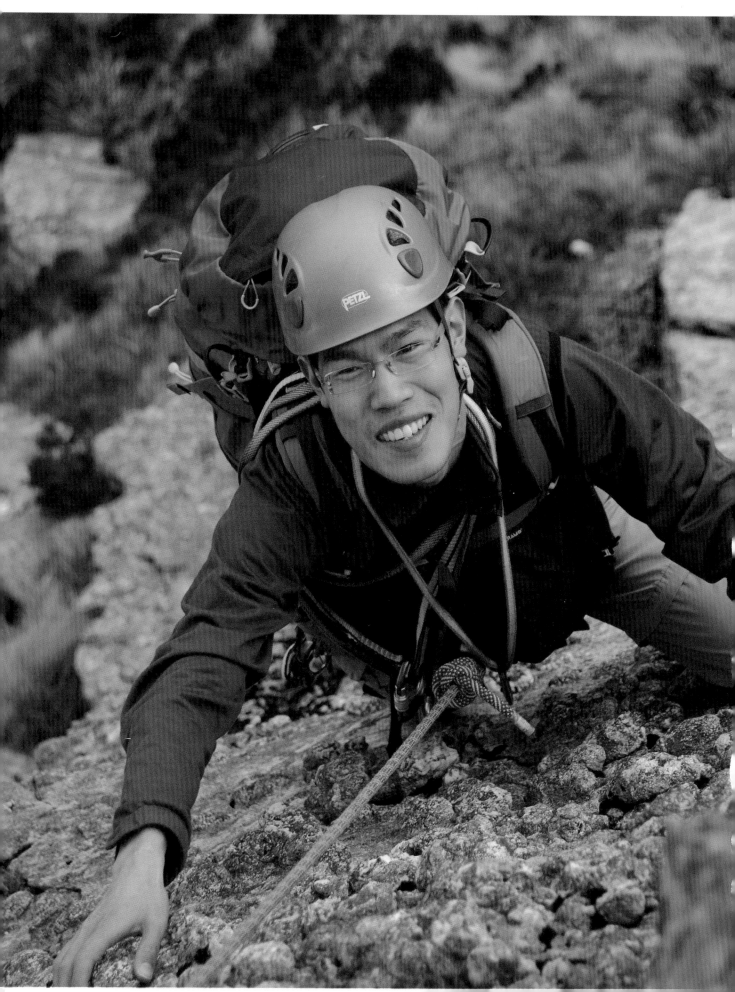

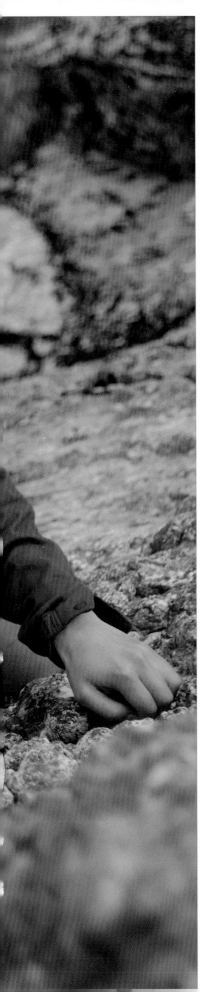

INTRODUCTION

A few years ago I met a guy climbing with his son on the sea cliffs in Pembrokeshire. In conversation it transpired that I had taught him to climb when he was a young man and that he had continued to climb ever since. He had introduced his own son to climbing and he had taken up the sport with a passion. It was quite possibly the most gratifying moment of my entire climbing career as an instructor and mountain guide.

This book is a distillation of the work that has made my life so rewarding. In these pages you'll not find the answers to everything you will ever need to know about rock climbing for it's a never-ending journey of discovery – not just about techniques – but also about yourself.

This book is more about inspiring you to have a go and take those first steps into the vertical world of the rock climber that may or may not lead to greater things. One of the finest attributes of climbing is the freedom it offers to express oneself and rather than be dogmatic and say that this is the way things must be done I have attempted to introduce techniques in a rather simplistic manner, relying heavily on photography of real climbers doing real climbing things. It's important to understand from the outset that there may be more than one way to achieve the same result. Similarly, the rope techniques required for safety are illustrated as uncluttered as is possible.

Any book of this nature may, at times, seem unfathomable. It is not a substitute for quality instruction from a qualified and experienced professional and I would urge anyone with a keen interest to seek out such tuition. This is particularly applicable to matters of safety where there is very little room for error or misunderstanding.

Most importantly of all, take care and enjoy yourself. If this book helps you to achieve those two things and you have a long and fruitful rock climbing adventure my job is done.

Nigel Shepherd
April 2014

BMC participation statement
"The BMC recognises that climbing, hill walking and mountaineering are activities with a danger of personal injury or death. Participants in these activities should be aware of and accept these risks and be responsible for their own actions and involvement."

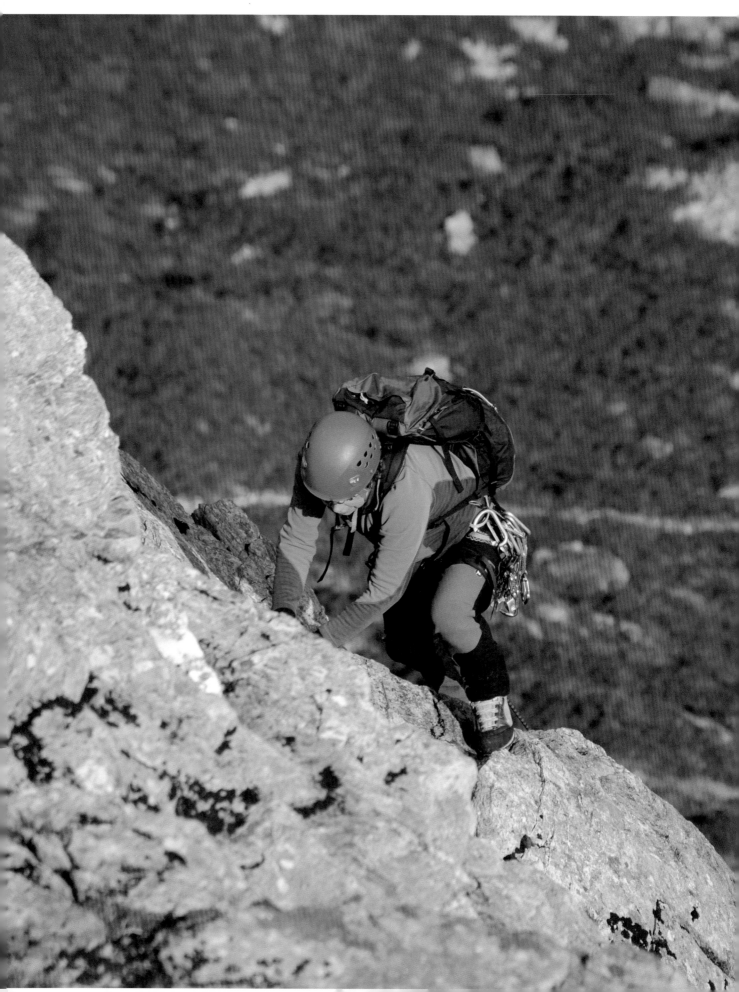

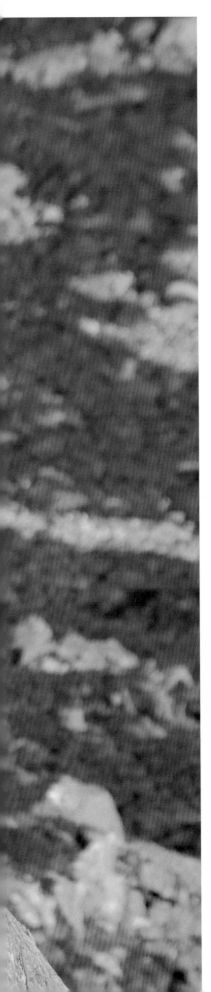

CHAPTER 1
WHY CLIMB?

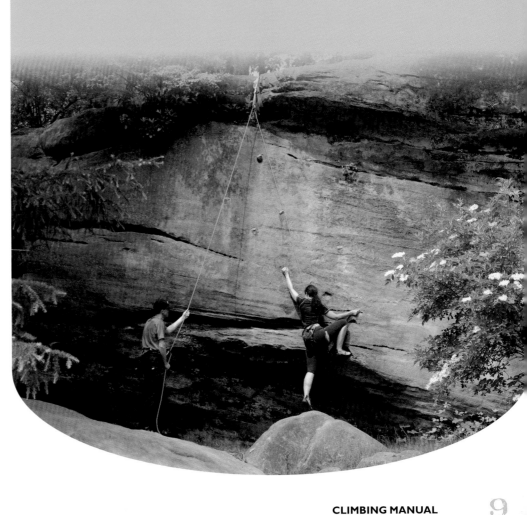

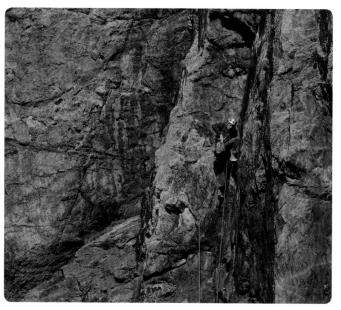

⬆ **Rock climbing is a unique sport offering physical activity with a degree of adventure.**

⬅ **A challenging climb will test experience, skill and bravery.**

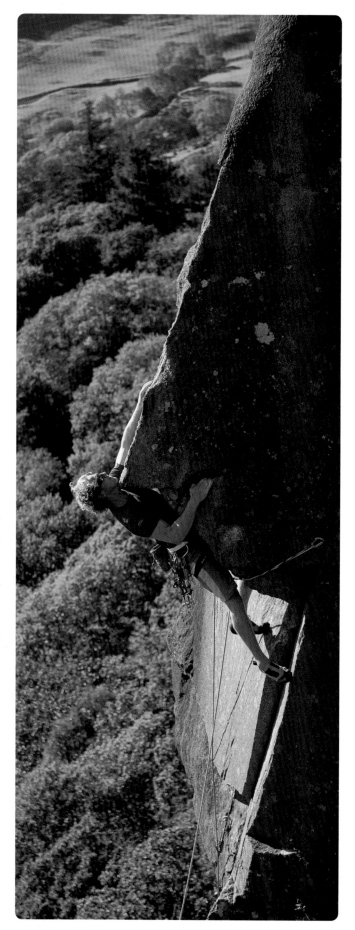

If you pose the question 'Why do you climb?' to a group of dedicated rock climbers you'll very likely glean a variety of responses from the romantic to verging on the slightly ridiculous. The mountaineer George Mallory famously responded with the answer, in reference to Everest, 'because it's there'. Dreamers may empathise with such a response but the practically minded will appreciate the more simplistic response coined by Tom Patey in an article entitled 'Apes or Ballerinas?'. Patey suggested that if every climber took time to consider Darwin and the Evolution of Man, the reason to climb would be obvious – because it's the natural thing to do.

I know why I go climbing and why I continue to enjoy the sport. I thrive on physical exercise and when I was still a youngster I was given opportunities to go to the hills to walk and to scramble. When I first tried rock climbing I was quite fearful and wasn't instantly sure that I'd like it very much. The people who had taken me under their wing in the hills were very encouraging. The breakthrough came when I was 16 and went on a climbing course based in Llanberis in North Wales. As I was by far the least experienced climber on the course, I found myself on some quite adventurous and difficult climbs. Though I was scared out of my wits for much of the time and seriously worn out at the end of each day, this was the catalyst that thrust me towards what, unknown to me at the time, would become my life. Within a year all I wanted to do was climb rocks!

At the time if you'd asked me why I'd become so fanatical about rock climbing I probably wouldn't have been able to give a satisfactory answer. I loved the physicality of it. I was a bit of a weedy lad at school, though good at gymnastics and long-distance running, and rock climbing gave me a great sense of physical satisfaction. As a youngster I was quite scared of heights but curiously rock climbing seemed not to bother me quite so much as teetering across an airy and narrow mountain ridge! And of course there was an element of danger and potential risk that spiced up the whole experience.

Nowadays the physicality is very challenging and I don't need quite so many risky situations to get my kicks. The fact that climbing can be gratifying at whatever level you choose makes it a uniquely challenging sport. Whether you're ambling up a long, gentle climb in the mountains on a sunny summer's day or cranking out difficult and technical climbing moves on a steep limestone wall, the immense satisfaction of success is the same sweet sensation.

Over the years my chosen pastime has given me the excuse needed to travel to far-off and exciting places. My first big rock-climbing trip was with a mate with whom I'd forged a strong climbing partnership and a great friendship. We were both 20 and had hatched a plan to go to North America for six months of climbing. The prospect of climbing continually for that long was too exciting for words and this was a truly memorable time, providing some wicked travelling and climbing adventures along the way. When you climb intensely like that for a long period you become very strong as well as technically more skilled thanks to such a concentrated period of practice. At times like those rock climbing is at its most joyous!

It's not all perfect though. There are times when rock climbing can be extremely frustrating. You may have set your sights on a particular climb and, for whatever reason, you try it and it doesn't come off. It might be because the conditions aren't ideal or the weather is poor, or the reason might be that you yourself aren't feeling on top form and everything is a struggle – the strength in your arms can wane alarmingly quickly and if your head isn't 'in the zone' it becomes more difficult to focus on what you need to do. There are many factors that might influence such frustrations. These things happen. They happen in all sports and they happen in life too I suppose. Such frustrations can be turned to positives on other days by mental application and careful planning. Mercifully such frustrating days are few.

One of the great aspects of rock climbing is the people you meet along the way: people you climb with and form friendships with, like-minded people whose aspirations are the same as yours, people who seek enjoyment and physical challenge in amazing surroundings without the distracting clutter of life's worries.

➡ **There's an abundance of moderately graded rock climbs offering plenty of fun and adventure in beautiful surroundings. This book will equip you with the skills to embark on a lifelong journey.**

⬇ **Climbing warm sun-kissed rock… in North Wales!**

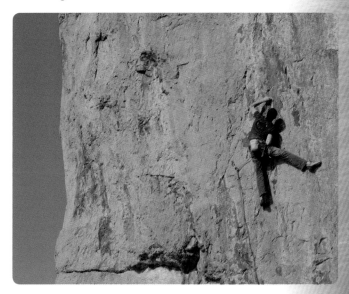

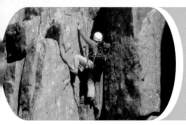

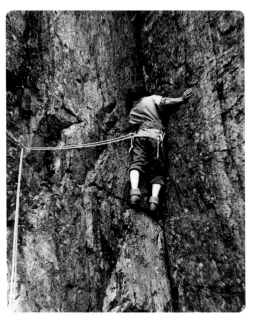

← In the early days climbing safety equipment was fairly rudimentary.

⬇ This photo of Main Wall, on a cliff called Cryn Las in the Snowdon massif of North Wales, illustrates the equipment available in the early 1950s.

→ Flying Buttress on Dinas Cromlech in the Llanberis Pass, North Wales, is a classic climb first ascended in 1931 by John Menlove Edwards. In this photo, taken around 1950, the leader has placed some very dubious protection around a dead tree branch.

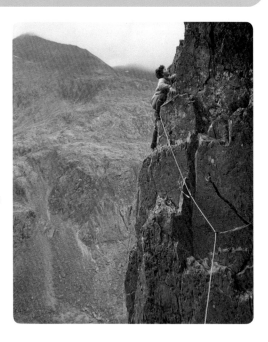

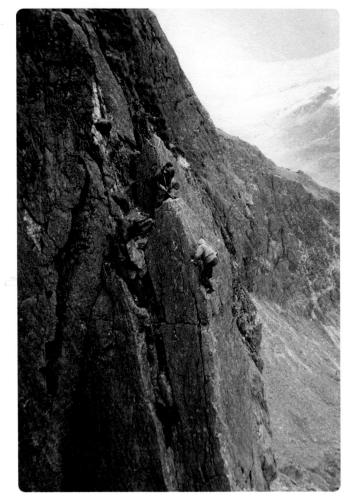

In the UK the ascent of Napes Needle on Great Gable in the Lake District is widely held to be the birth of the sport. In truth, climbers had been making ascents of easy rocky ridges and gullies for many years but in 1886 a group led by W.P. Haskett Smith climbed the Napes purely 'for sport' and their adventure captured the attention of mountaineers. To this day this is still a moderately testing climb and the top of the pinnacle has barely sufficient space to accommodate two climbers.

At the time of the first ascent of the Napes and through the following two or three decades, rock climbing was potentially an extremely dangerous sport. The first person (the leader) to climb up had to rely purely on skill and a steady nerve along with strength to grip to the rock face. Once up a section of rock, the leader would then be able to bring up his compatriots on a rope by standing braced and securing the rope around his shoulder. Ropes were made of hemp or sisal and of indeterminate breaking strength! Occasionally, if the situation demanded, climbers would form human pyramids to overcome a difficult obstacle and once one was up the remaining members of the party could be hoisted upwards on the rope! During this period of evolution of the sport the mantra for all climbers was that 'the leader must never fall'.

Through the early part of the 20th century climbers began to explore more difficult and unlikely lines of ascent up cliffs, with innovative techniques for protecting the leader. One example was to use a piece of rope threaded around a large rock jammed in a crack (a chokestone or chockstone) and then tied to enclose the climbing rope, and, similarly, a rope could be looped over a spike of rock and tied to encircle the climbing rope. In the late 1920s Fred Pigott climbed a series of stepped cracks on the cliff of Clogwyn Du'r Arddu in Snowdonia, North Wales, and carried with him several round pebbles of varying size that he jammed in narrow cracks with a thinner rope (sling) threaded around them, and then attached the rope using a steel karabiner. This was the very first time such a system of safeguarding a climb was used and it's the basis for all climbing safety to this day – though Pigott would be astounded at how sophisticated and technical climbing protection has become.

The boundaries of what might be humanly possible on steeper and more improbable-looking cliffs were continually being pushed. During the 1950s climbing took a huge leap forward technically, in terms of both what could be climbed and the use of safety protection. In one other respect that decade also marked a very significant turning point in mountain sport generally. During the late 19th and early 20th centuries the climbing fraternity was largely the preserve of the well-off, including aristocrats with time on their hands and money to spend on lavish holidays in the mountains of the UK and abroad. After the Second World War this changed dramatically and within a few years climbing became a sport for all.

One well-known name among the new generation led the way with a different attitude to climbing. Joe Brown, along with equally talented climbing companions, not only pushed the difficulty of what could be climbed but also explored and pioneered new climbs on faces that were hitherto deemed blank and devoid of holds. Brown and his compatriots also devised ways to use crack protection to greater effect. Instead of carrying pebbles to be jammed into cracks and threaded, these talented and courageous climbers used engineering nuts threaded on slings made of newly available nylon rope. It's rumoured that the first nuts used in this way were taken from the sleepers of the railway up Snowdon!

By the early 1960s the first commercially available chockstones were being made. The very first of these was called the Acorn, which bore very little resemblance to the drilled-out nuts previously used. This was soon followed by the MOAC, a wedge-shaped nut threaded with rope. By the start of the 1970s the floodgates were opening and all manner of shapes and sizes began to appear, some threaded with wire, others with nylon cord. The effect this development was to have on climbing standards and safety proved to be profound. Along with the use of nylon ropes and the introduction of climbing harnesses, the three decades following the 1950s were the most intense and significant period in the short time that rock climbing has been considered a worthy sport.

The latter decades of the 20th century also brought other significant developments. Special climbing shoes with smooth but sticky rubber soles allowed better adhesion to the rock. Leader-protection devices made a huge leap with the invention of 'Friends' by American climber Ray Jardine. Still manufactured to this day, these devices feature four independently operating cams that are spring-loaded and open out inside a crack to bite into the rock. In all their various forms, from the tiniest through to the most enormous, 'Friends' provide crack protection in places where 25 years ago it couldn't have been considered.

From the 1970s through to the early part of the 21st century, climbing standards were consolidated and pushed forward at the same time, with more climbers climbing hard but equally some super-talented climbers pushing the grades to the very limits of conceivability. This mix of consolidation with a push for ever-higher standards continues to evolve to this day. As always, those pushing the limits are few and highly skilled, but nowadays there are far greater numbers performing at a high level than ever before.

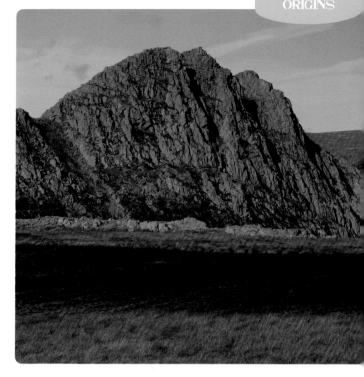

⬆ **The East Face of Tryfan, where many climbs were first made in the 1800s. Today, it's a popular trad climbing area with climbs of up to 150m in length and a good, stiff walk to reach them.**

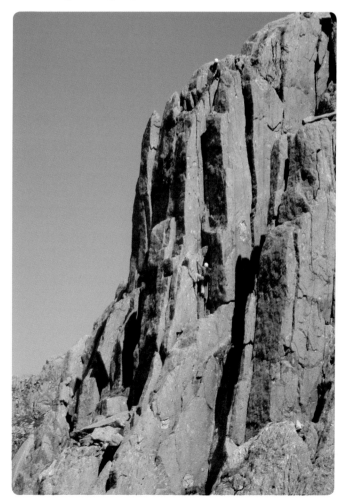

➡ **Direct Route on Glyder Fach in Snowdonia is another classic climb, typical of the era around 1900; following a line of obvious weakness up a seemingly improbable face.**

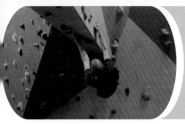
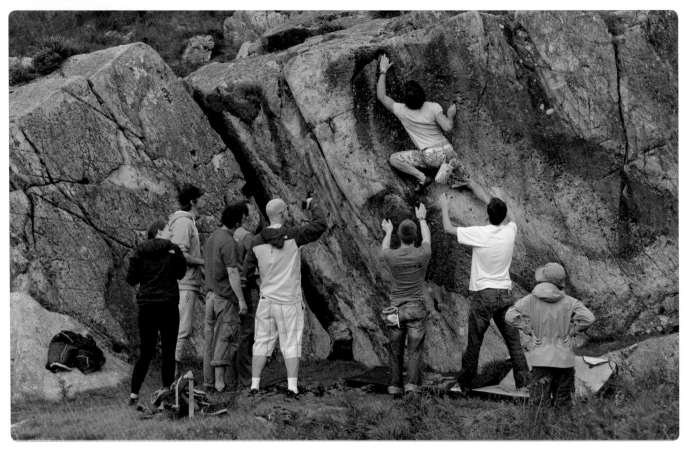

↑ **Bouldering has rapidly become a sport in its own right. Climbers have always embraced the concept of climbing short but challenging problems, largely as a means to train but also for fun and as a social activity, but with the advent of bouldering mats it has blossomed into a great sport with a dedicated following.**

In earlier times, if you climbed rock you were simply deemed to be a rock climber, with all aspects of the sport encompassed within that single nomenclature. Nowadays, however, rock climbing is more complex and the sport is split into sub-categories; one can choose to focus on a single category or embrace all categories for the full experience!

BOULDERING

This is pure rock climbing. It focuses on working out a sequence of moves to overcome a relatively short section of climbing on boulders.

Boulder problems can be very short, with no more than three or four moves close to the ground, or slightly longer when higher above the ground. To increase the length of a boulder problem, climbers will often create traverse climbs where climbing continues around a boulder or across a small cliff face. Bouldering doesn't normally require the use of ropes or technical equipment, though some higher problems, known as 'highballs', can benefit from a rope,

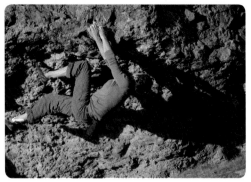

← **Many boulder problems are only a short distance above the ground.**

especially with difficult or treacherous landings below if one had to jump off.

The tools for bouldering are a pair of climbing shoes, a chalk bag and a crash pad or mat. The intensity of difficulty achieved in the best bouldering in the world is incredible. Many of the hardest problems are intractable on a cliff high above the ground using ropes and other safety equipment – though, it has to be said, this is where standards will advance to eventually.

Rock climbers have traditionally used bouldering as a form of training for climbing but there are growing numbers for whom it's a sport in its own right.

INDOOR CLIMBING

The impact of indoor venues on the development of climbing cannot be underestimated. This has manifested itself in a number of positive ways for the sport. Primarily it has allowed many thousands more people the opportunity to sample the sport unfettered by weather, season or location. Equally significantly, it has contributed to a huge number of climbers improving their standards. Until the 1980s, the number of climbers around the world climbing at the more extreme grades could be numbered in hundreds, but nowadays there are many thousands.

Climbing walls have evolved to become sporting destinations in their own right and there are many people who only climb indoors – and to a very high standard. For many, though, a climbing wall is an ideal stepping stone to outdoor climbing, while for those who already have outdoor rock experience it offers the best training environment during the winter months. Indoor climbing on walls is a low-risk activity compared with 'trad climbing' outdoors and allows the climber to focus on skill development in an ideal environment without distractions.

Alongside the development of climbing walls as a means to train, the coaching of climbing to achieve more efficient movement has also taken off. Training regimes have become a significant part of any serious climber's programme. Long gone are the times when a day of hard climbing had to be followed by a hard night's drinking!

If you climb only indoors you need a bare minimum of climbing equipment – climbing shoes, chalk bag, harness, belay device and screwgate karabiner. If you want to lead climbs, you'll also need a rope. Many climbing wall venues will offer taster sessions to those who'd like to try climbing as well as a series of learning and progression sessions for beginners.

On climbing walls the rope is used to safeguard the climber and this is done in one of two ways, as follows.

- A rope is fixed at the top of a climb, often permanently, and the climber ties on to one end of it while the other end is secured through a belay device held by a second person. As the climber moves up the wall the second person takes in the slack rope through the device; these devices are designed so that if you have to hold a falling climber you can do so easily (see Chapter 6 for more detail). After reaching the top the climber is then lowered back down on the rope by the second person.
- The second method is called 'leading'. The two climbers start with the rope on the ground. The person who will go up first ties on to the end of the rope. The second person takes the rope and threads it through the belay device. The leader climbs up the wall clipping into karabiners attached to fixed anchors at regular intervals (these are called 'quickdraws'). If the leader falls it's hoped that a combination of these fixed anchors and the second person holding the rope through a belay device will arrest the fall. In theory the leading climber can only fall twice the distance that he or she is above the fixed anchor. This is a simple outline of the whole procedure and it's covered in considerably more detail in Chapter 7.

SPORT CLIMBING

This style of climbing is rather like indoor climbing but takes place outside on real rock. It's probably the most popular style of rock climbing around the world.

There are many reasons why sport climbing is so popular but the two that stand out most are its very low level of risk and the fact that it can be experienced in some stunningly beautiful locations. It's safer than trad climbing (see below) because all protection for the

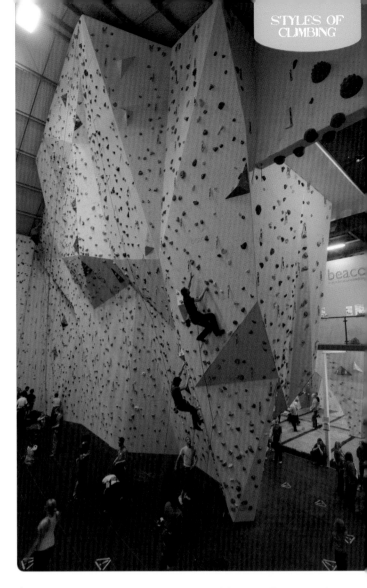

⬆ **Indoor climbing walls offer the prospect of climbing all year round and are ideal venues for taking your first steps into the vertical world as well as for developing further as a climber.**

⬇ **Bouldering indoors is intense, and a great way to develop skills, strength and endurance.**

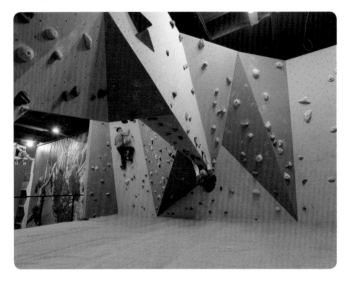

Sport climbing is the most natural progression from indoors to outdoors and takes place all around the world in some amazingly beautiful locations. Protection by pre-fixed bolt anchors provides a comforting sense of safety and a minimum amount of kit is required.

lead climber is by means of bolts that are drilled and fixed into the rock face. These are solid anchor points and, if placed at regular and sensible intervals, afford comforting protection for the leader, knowing that a fall should result in a safe ending! (There are, of course, some very 'sporting' sport routes where this may not be the case and these should be considered and approached with the same attitude you would adopt for trad climbing.)

Many sport climbs are of a single-pitch variety where the climber ascends for less than half the length of the rope and then returns to the ground. Around the world there are also multi-pitch sport climbs, some of which are hundreds of metres long and may take a day or more to ascend.

For sport climbing you'll need harness, climbing shoes, belay device, a couple of screwgate karabiners, chalk bag, a set of quickdraws and a rope.

While sport climbing can be done on all manner of rock types, including granite and slate, it is most prevalent on limestone, where naturally occurring cracks and fissures are absent from seemingly smooth and compact faces.

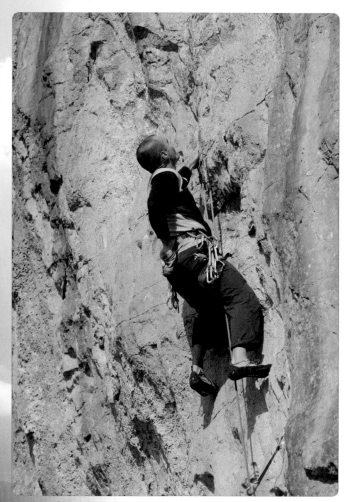

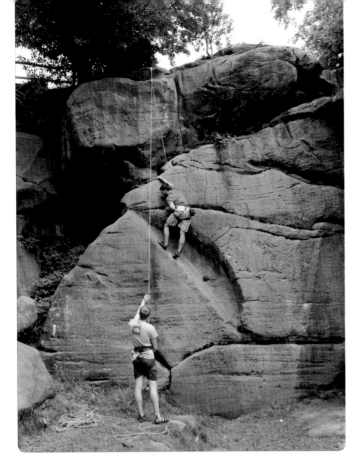

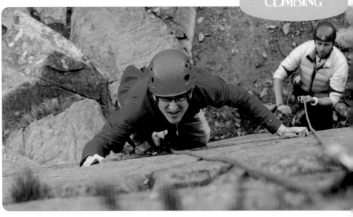

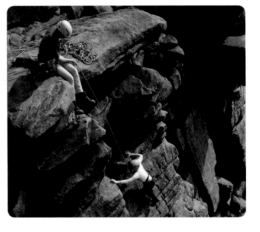

⬆ Bottom roping on sandstone in southern England: the anchor is fixed at the top and the climbing rope clipped to it to form a pulley system; the climber is safeguarded by a companion who belays the rope; on sandstone outcrops like this, the climber must go over the top of the climb before untying from the rope and throwing it back down.

⬆ Bottom roping is a great way to learn. The security of a rope from above, the companionship of friends and colleagues egging you on all conspire to create a comfortable learning environment.

➡ Top roping is where the belayer will walk or scramble around to the top of a short crag, anchor himself, and then bring the climber up to the top using a belaying technique.

⬇ A short piece of rock of low angle is an ideal place to introduce young children to rock climbing.

⬇ Not a beginner's climb by any means, but bottom roping at crags can also be used to help develop strength and technique.

SINGLE-PITCH TOP ROPING OR BOTTOM ROPING

This is a style of climbing adopted by instructors or outdoor centres where a short outcrop of rock is used to introduce beginners to the sport. There's no reason why, given some basic rope skills, any group of climbers couldn't set up a similar climbing scenario in order to gain experience. In fact it's an excellent way to master the techniques of anchor placement and construction, and to practise belaying skills.

To set up for top or bottom roping, you need first to go around to the top of the outcrop and rig an anchor. This is sometimes done using a separate rope from the climbing rope, by linking together a number of anchors and then having a central attachment point draped over the edge of the outcrop, with a climbing rope doubled through it and attached using a screwgate karabiner. Both rope ends are dropped down the crag and the climber climbs up on one end while the belayer safeguards the other through a belay device. This is widely known as bottom roping and is very similar to climbing at an indoor venue using fixed ropes.

An alternative is to sit the belayer at the top of the outcrop and attach him to the anchor points so that he can't be pulled over the edge. A climber ties on to the rope end, which is safeguarded by the belayer at the top of the crag. This is called top roping.

There are some climbing crags or outcrops where bottom roping is the only permitted way to climb. The sandstone outcrops found in southern England are an example. This style is adopted to help prevent erosion of relatively 'soft' rock.

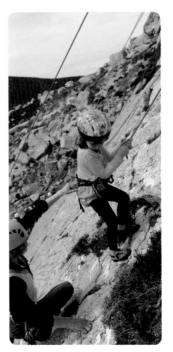

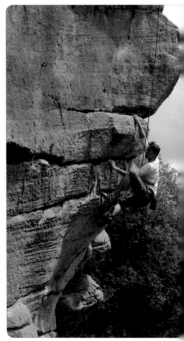

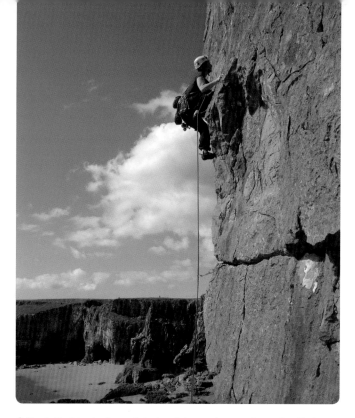

TRAD CLIMBING

This style of climbing has its roots firmly in the finest traditions of the sport and has flourished since the very earliest days of the pioneering climbers of the 19th century. Trad climbing demands a particular approach based on the premise of self-sufficiency in terms of skill and safety as well as the requirement that climbers leave no trace of their passing. As such it carries a higher level of risk and sometimes a more uncertain outcome than the styles already covered. This adventure approach is the very essence of trad climbing.

A team for trad climbing is normally two climbers or quite often three, but more than three will significantly slow down proceedings. The team will arrive at the bottom of a cliff and climb up it using a recognised route; the cliff will have a name, a description in a guidebook and a grade for the level of seriousness of the route. If the climb is longer than the length of rope allows, it will be climbed in a series of stages called pitches. The leader will ascend a pitch, placing protection in cracks or around flakes of rock while the second climber holds the leader's rope in a belay device. On arriving at the top of a pitch the leader arranges anchors to secure to and then brings up the second climber. The whole process is repeated until the top of the climb is reached.

A short multi-pitch climb will consist of two pitches but around the globe there are climbs of more than 30 pitches that can take many days to ascend.

⬆ **Trad climbing is the real deal and demands more from the climber in terms of understanding how to climb safely. The rewards are there for the taking.**

⬇ **Fine trad climbing just a short bus ride from Sheffield! Stanage Edge in Derbyshire is one of myriad gritstone outcrops found all over the Peak District and Yorkshire Dales National Parks. Many of the most celebrated climbers began their adventures on crags like this.**

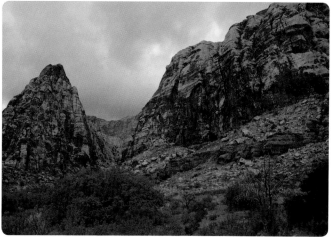

⬆⬇ **Multi-pitch trad climbing takes place on crags that are much longer than the length of a climbing rope and climbers ascend in stages, known as pitches; the second photo here zooms in on climbers high on the face.**

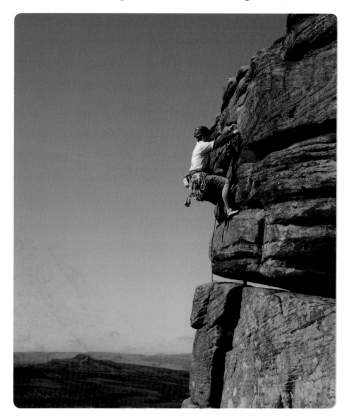

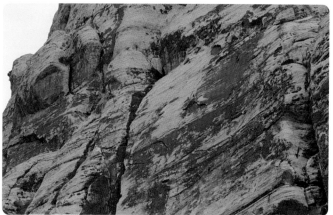

There are ethical standards, unwritten but accepted by all who climb, handed down from generation to generation. These are simple enough and can be summarised in two ways:

▨ Don't damage or deface the rock.
▨ Don't resort to artificial aids to gain advantage.

The equipment required for trad climbing is significantly more varied than for sport climbing. The climbers will need to arrange their own protection as they ascend, by placing wedge, hexagonal or camming devices into cracks in the rock face. Sizes and shapes of crack vary enormously and so a number of different sizes of crack protection must be carried. More difficult climbs that ascend blanker faces may require very small, thin crack protection whereas the easier climbs will commonly utilise larger pieces of protection. The skills required to place protection are covered in detail in Chapter 5.

OTHER STYLES OF CLIMBING

Solo climbing is where the climber goes out alone and without equipment with which to arrange protection. Solo climbing is the most dangerous of all climbing styles and carries a high risk of death or serious injury if you fall. Often non-climbers incorrectly use the term 'free climbing' for solo climbing, but the proper definition of free climbing is where the climber doesn't use artificially created handholds or footholds to gain advantage during the ascent.

One form of solo climbing where a fall could be less serious is deep water soloing (DWS). Climbs are commonly no more than 10 metres high but there are plenty that are higher. The accepted practice is to climb the route and then jump off from the top or just below the top. There are recognised areas around the coast of the UK where DWS takes place and there are many areas abroad.

Big-wall climbing is a style of climbing on huge rock faces that may take several days to ascend and may require the use of artificial aids to overcome sections of blankness on the wall. Climbers will sleep on the rock face and carry all food and water for the ascent with them

Cenotaph Corner in North Wales, first climbed by Joe Brown and climbing partner Doug Belshaw in 1952, is one of the world's most famous and recognisable climbs; in this photo the climbers are on Left Wall, a later addition to the wall and one that has become a benchmark of its grade.

in bags that are hauled up behind them as they go. Where no ledges are available to sleep on, they will sleep in hammocks suspended from the wall.

That, then, is an overview of the sport of rock climbing. It's not totally exhaustive by any means, but an understanding of the roots of the sport means we can launch off into the nitty-gritty of what we need to learn to take those first steps…

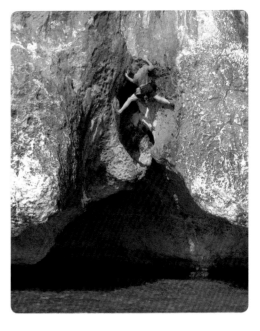

➜ **Deep water soloing – chalk bag and climbing shoes are all that's needed, along with deep water below the crag. If you want to do more than one climb you'll need plenty of chalk bags.**

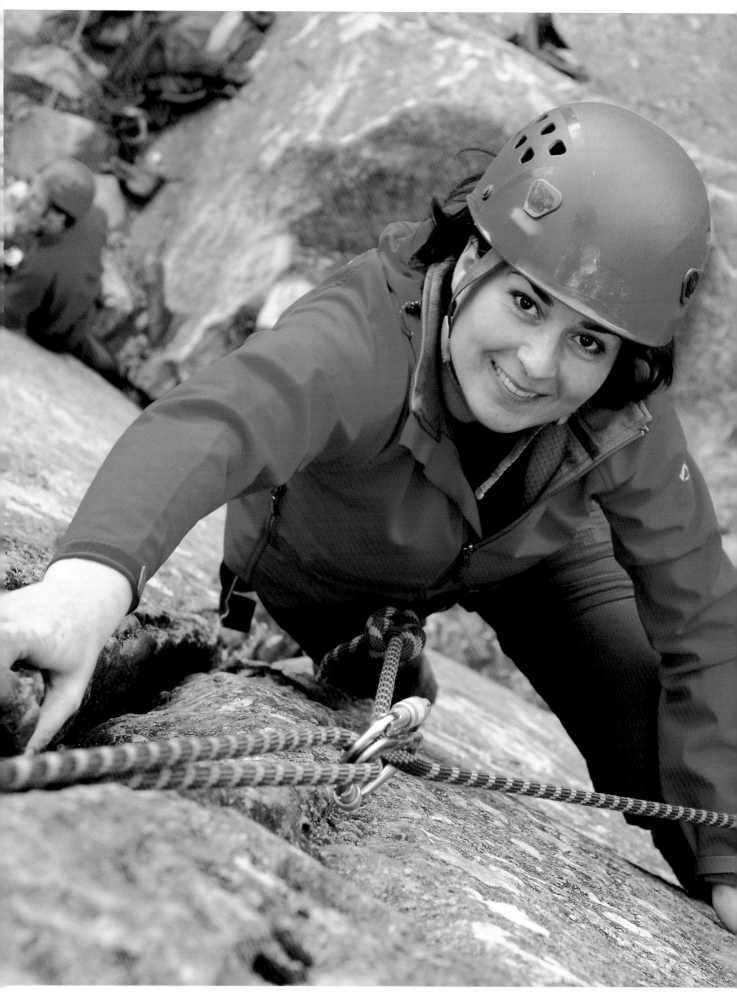

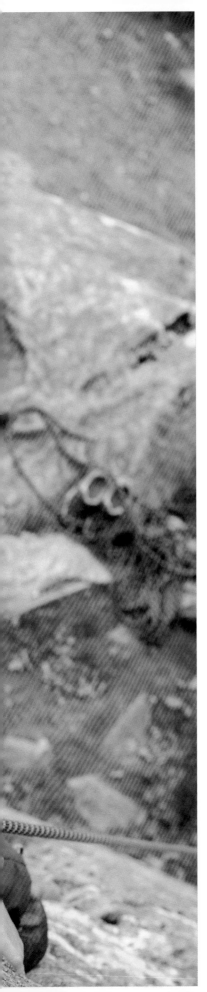

CHAPTER 2

GETTING STARTED

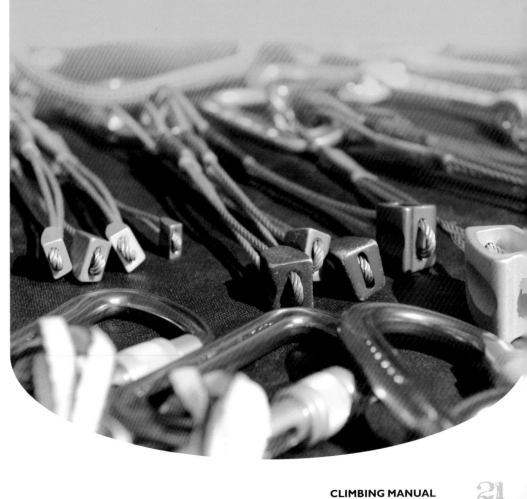

Two of the very first questions asked by people who are considering rock climbing are 'Am I too old?' and 'I don't think I have the strength to hang on'. Both are genuine concerns but needn't cause any problems.

Provided that you're fairly physically able, you can never be too old to try the sport. Many years ago I introduced a man in his 50s to rock climbing. He loved it from the moment he set foot on the rock and climbed for two decades before having to give up due to failing health. He never climbed particularly difficult routes but he achieved a good standard and was able to climb some of the classic ascents in the UK and Europe.

You do need some strength in your hands and arms to climb but surprisingly little if you choose low-angled rock faces. The basis of good climbing technique lies with footwork. If you're able to use your feet well and take most of your weight over footholds, there are innumerable climbs you could do – easily more than a lifetime's worth!

Another concern frequently voiced is a fear of heights. This is a genuine and sometimes worrying fear but it's not insurmountable. Being tied into a rope that's securely anchored will go some considerable way to allaying fears. So too will the fact that when you climb your height above the ground increases only gradually, giving you time to accustom yourself to the feeling. Of course there are people for whom height is a truly unnerving experience and overcoming it may not be possible.

If you have friends or family who climb already and are keen to take you climbing, either indoors or outdoors, this is the most 'traditional' way to start. You may have a background of hillwalking and scrambling with them and already have some idea of what climbing might be like. Going out with a trusted and experienced friend or family member will help to put you at your ease immediately and they'll certainly have your best interests at heart. If you choose to take this course as an introduction to the sport it's vital that appropriate levels of difficulty are considered and acted on. It's not much fun being introduced to climbing if the climb you're attempting is far too difficult or steep for you. An over-zealous 'baptism by fire' at the hardest end of the spectrum is not to be recommended! An ideal outdoors venue would be a low-angled slab of rock with good anchors at the top and plenty of open space at the bottom; something around 10m in height is perfect.

The other, and possibly better, option is to join one of the many courses of instruction run by qualified rock climbing instructors or mountain guides. Those qualified to teach climbing undergo considerable

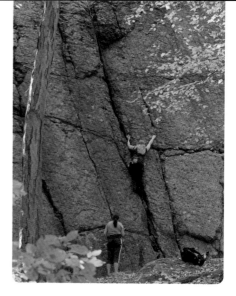

→ **A short, simple climb is an ideal place to experience climbing for the first time.**

training and assessment and are not only committed rock climbers in their spare time but also passionate about encouraging novices.

Courses, whether indoors or outdoors, will follow a structured progression that will normally begin with movement on rock – how to use feet and hands both for balance and for grip (see Chapter 3). This will be followed by a look at the basic equipment, how to tie on to the rope and how to safeguard each other using the rope, and finally putting it all together on a climb or two.

Indoor climbing venues offer introductory sessions that are structured over a number of visits, usually lasting an hour or two at a time. Some indoor venues offer longer courses that will also include a visit to an outdoor crag if the weather is suitable. Courses are also available that last a whole week, by the end of which you may even get to lead your own climbs under strict supervision. Obviously such courses give you an opportunity to learn even more about the sport, particularly in terms of safety procedures.

A big advantage of attending a course is that you'll be provided with all the equipment you need, so at least you'll have a good idea of whether or not you're likely to continue climbing before you part with hard-earned cash.

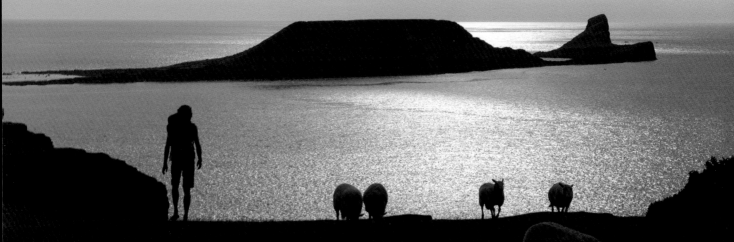

Approaching a climb may involve a simple walk or a much longer mountain walk.

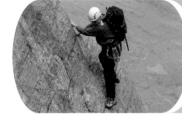

CLOTHING

You don't necessarily need to buy any special clothing when you're starting out – something sporty and hard-wearing that doesn't restrict movement is perfectly fine. Having said that, there's a vast array of outdoor clothing available and there'll certainly be a style and colour to suit all tastes. There have been some fairly wacky fashion trends over the years!

The most important considerations are to make sure that clothing fits well, allows for flexible movement and is hard-wearing; light fabrics don't take to being rubbed against rough rock!

Base layer could be a cotton T-shirt but it may be more comfortable to use a specific outdoor base layer that provides wicking and insulating properties. I'm a great fan of merino wool, which isn't as itchy as it sounds and provides warmth if required, but is also fairly cool when used just as a T-shirt.

Fleece sweaters or jackets are by far the most efficient tops to wear. Made entirely of man-made fibres, they provide an essential warm layer, particularly when covered by a windproof shell. Legwear is commonly either man-made fabric or a mix of cotton canvas and harder-wearing man-made fabrics.

Other considerations may include the seasons for your climbing: do you want to keep warm on chilly days or cool on hot days? It isn't vital for clothing to keep you dry in the rain because you probably won't often climb outdoors in wet weather, and if you do you'll need waterproof 'shell' clothing. You may want protection from wind chill, as even a light breeze on a moderately warm day can cool you down rapidly if you're belaying or waiting to climb. A lightweight insulating jacket is ideal for belaying work

at sport climbing venues and may be essential on a cool autumn or winter day. Add to that a lightweight windproof shell and you're clothed for most spring, summer or early autumn conditions.

Footwear for approaching the crags you'll climb depends very much on the length and type of walk necessary to reach the crag. In most instances a pair of sturdy trainers will suffice. If you have to walk further you may choose to wear a pair of 'approach shoes'. These are much more substantial than training shoes, usually providing a rugged sole and a little more support than trainers. Some styles also feature 'sticky' rubber soles that are suited to simple climbing. Very occasionally, climbers might approach a crag wearing hillwalking or mountain boots, but this is more relevant to remote crags requiring a long approach walk.

If it's really chilly, rock climbing can be quite unpleasant, but it's certainly made more comfortable if you have gloves and a woolly hat. If it's so cold that you feel the need to climb with gloves on, do your climbing indoors or go home to a cosy fire.

A backpack is also required to carry all your kit to the crag. There's such a plethora of packs and designs on the market that it would be impossible to cover all the detail here. What you'll need is something around 25–35 litres in capacity and ideally a fairly 'technical' pack, in that it's designed to be comfortable when carrying a fair amount of weight for reasonably long approaches.

As well as climbing gear, you'll most likely need to carry some spare clothing and food and drink. It's also a good idea to have a small first-aid kit in your backpack.

⬇ **Shorts and T-shirt are comfortable clothing for warm days – be prepared for scratched knees though.**

⬇ **Long pants designed to be hard wearing and with articulated knees for freedom of movement are essential wear for most climbing. If you want to climb in jeans, don't expect to be able to move freely – unless they are a stretchy variety. A chalk bag is carried on a strap around the waist.**

⬇ **A simple backpack will suffice for a short walk to a crag, but if you climb on high mountain crags you may need to carry a backpack on your climb so a slightly more technically orientated design is preferable.**

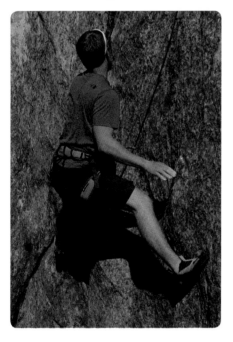

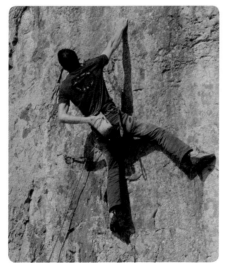

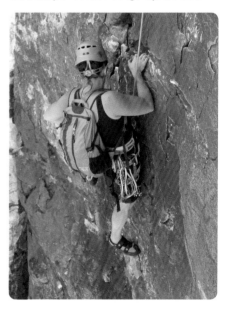

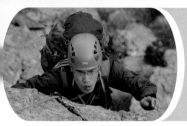
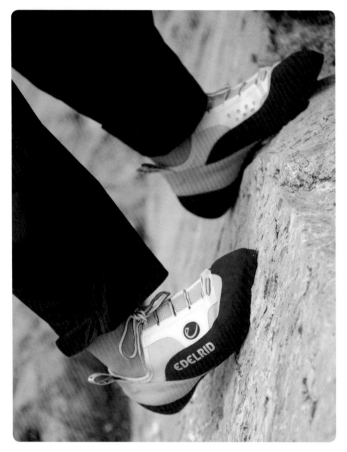

⬆ **A comfortable all-round shoe of the lace-up variety; shoes such as this are comfortable to wear for long periods. When you begin there's no need to cram your feet into ridiculously tight-fitting shoes.**

⬇ **A technical shoe with a hook-and-loop fastening system such as this one needs to be worn quite tight – maybe even one or two sizes smaller than normal. Such shoes are normally only worn when actually climbing and immediately removed on returning to the ground; for the novice climber, however, the close precision of such a shoe offers little advantage.**

CLIMBING SHOES

At first sight climbing shoes may appear slightly alien. Like strangely shaped trainers, they look incredibly uncomfortable and they have no tread on the soles. But look further and you'll soon see that they're designed for a purpose.

Soles of climbing shoes are made from soft rubber that's intended to stick to dry rock. The rubber adheres to smooth rock but also takes advantage of any irregularities in the rock surface to mould itself around protuberances. The overall effect is one of superb grip. The sticky rubber band that encircles the upper shoe and the toe will also give added grip when the boot is wedged within a crack or with the side up against rock.

The closure system is either Velcro or laces. There are advantages to both: Velcro is quickly adjusted and easily undone when you need to take off the shoes; laces offer fine adjustment to provide a closer fit around the whole foot. Manufacturers also offer slipper-style climbing shoes and these are designed to be worn quite tightly. The boot needs to wrap snugly around your foot so that when you stand sideways on a foothold the shoe won't roll around your foot; similarly the heel should be fairly secure in the boot. To this end rock shoes are shaped to a greater or lesser extent.

There are particular styles of shoe that are better suited to certain types of climbing than others. When starting out you'll benefit from having a shoe that fits well but errs slightly on the comfortable side. Climbers at the very top of their game may choose to wear extremely tight-fitting shoes, as small as two sizes below normal foot size! Add to that the radical curvature in the shape of the shoe and as a beginner your initial impression – that climbing footwear resembles some form of ancient Chinese torture – will only be reinforced. Such shoes may be so excruciatingly uncomfortable that you cease to see the point of climbing at all!

Most shoes leave your ankle bones exposed, though there are a few boot-style designs that give a little protection from cuts and scrapes on the ankles.

⬇ **The La Sportiva Katana is an excellent shoe that can be worn tightly or as a comfortable fit; the lace-up version allows fine adjustment around the foot.**

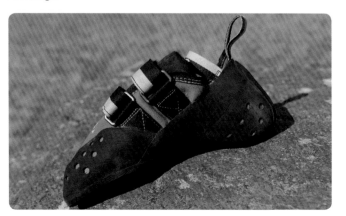

As a beginner it's best to start with a style of shoe that's comfortable, not too radically shaped and doesn't pinch your toes, and then change to a more technical shoe when you have gained some experience.

If you have an opportunity to try different styles and makes of shoes while on a climb, then you'll at least have an advantage when it comes to buying your first pair of shoes. Without that opportunity it's important to spend time trying on different makes and styles in-store to find the shoe that suits you best.

HARNESS

Climbers wear a harness so that when they're hanging on a rope, or if they fall, it's a comfortable experience – or at least as comfortable as can be expected. If climbing shoes present a bewildering choice, harness types may confuse even more.

Rock-climbing harnesses are made up of two parts – the waist belt and the leg loops. The leg loops are linked to the waist belt by a very strong sewn loop referred to as the 'belay loop' (or sometimes 'abseil loop'). At the rear the leg loops are normally attached to the underside of the waist belt by means of an adjustable elastic strap. (There are harnesses that don't feature a belay loop but these are intended for more general mountaineering purposes rather than pure rock climbing).

There are two main types of harness – fixed leg loop and adjustable leg loop – and within these alternatives there are also various styles as well as specific designs for men and women. Your choice depends on what sort of climbing you expect to do.

For indoor climbing and sports climbing a harness with fixed leg loops and a lightly padded waistband will be perfectly adequate. The waist belt should feature at least three or four gear loops to which essential bits of kit can be clipped. For trad climbing, where you may have a considerable amount of hardware dangling from the waist belt of the harness, you need to consider a harness with a more substantial waist belt and a greater number of gear loops to support and accommodate the extra weight.

Fitting a harness correctly is essential. The waist belt is exactly what it says it is – it should fit around the waist and above the hips. When you tighten and secure the locking buckle, there should be at least 10cm of webbing strap to spare. The leg loops should fit snugly but not tightly around the upper thighs, and the rise between the leg loops and the waist should be comfortably accommodated by the belay loop.

If the available combinations of fixed leg loops and waist belt don't provide a good fit, then take the option of a harness with adjustable leg loops. If you think that the circumference of your upper thighs might vary considerably in the future, then always take this option!

A note of caution: very small children have a lower centre of gravity than adults and also their hips aren't fully formed. If you're buying a harness for a child you should consider one that incorporates a chest

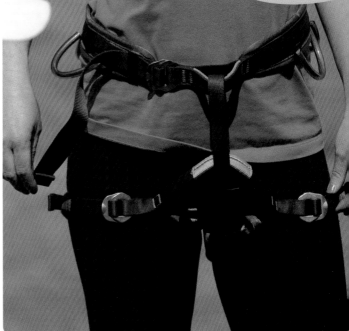

↑ **A climbing harness is made up of waist belt and leg loops that are connected by a strong sewn loop called the belay loop. The buckle to secure the waist belt is called a 'ziplock' and is easily adjusted but never completely undone. The spare webbing can be tucked into securing loops on the belt itself. When you size up a harness, the correct fit is achieved with the waist belt around the waist with a minimum of 8cm spare tail on the adjustment strap. Adjustable leg loops are a great idea, though fixed-size leg-loop harnesses are also available for a small weight and cost saving.**

harness; this is called a full-body harness and the attachment point is at sternum level rather than waist level.

The method for tying a climbing rope into a harness is determined by the manufacturer of the particular harness. Though most harnesses follow the same principle, there are some that differ. Follow the manufacturer's recommendations to the letter when tying in to the rope (see Chapter 4).

↖↓ **Another style of buckle closure is one that must be threaded back on itself for security. If not threaded back, the slippage of the buckle is dangerously low – only a few kilos rather than several tonnes.**

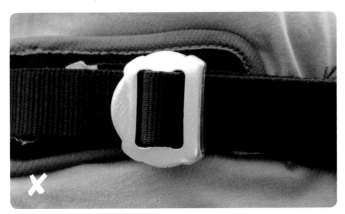

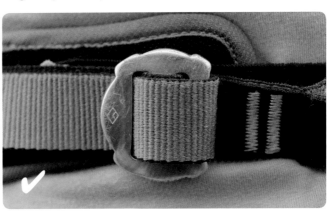

← Small stones at the top of a crag or cliff form just one of many potential hazards that more than justify the wearing of a helmet. A beginner should always wear a helmet; once you gain experience you can make your own choice about whether to continue wearing one.

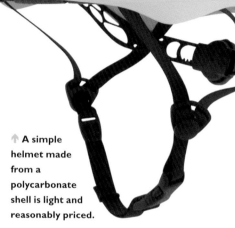

↑ A simple helmet made from a polycarbonate shell is light and reasonably priced.

⬇ A simple helmet-adjustment dial: the advantage with this type of adjustment is that it can be altered while the helmet is worn.

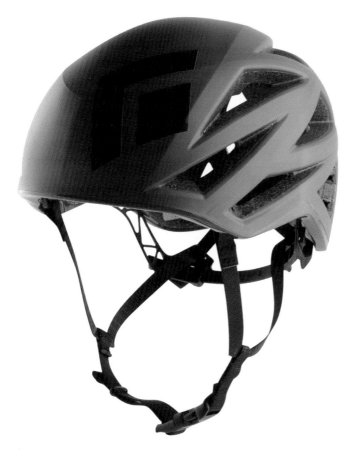

⬆ **A superlight helmet is ideal for wearing and carrying on longer days out on the crags.**

CLIMBING HELMET

Safety equipment manufacturers must conform to international standards set by the UIAA (Union Internationale des Associations d'Alpinisme) and equipment for sale in the European Union must conform to PPE (Personal Protective Equipment) regulation for each individual type of product, but there isn't any official governing body to regulate rock climbing as a sport and therefore no obligations on participants in the sport to abide by any rules.

It isn't compulsory, therefore, to wear a helmet, though of course it's very sensible to do so, no matter how experienced you are. There are climbers who never wear a helmet, citing the distraction it causes or how hot they get in warm sunshine, but it makes no sense to try to justify not wearing a helmet.

A stone the size of a gobstopper dislodged from 100m above will do some very nasty damage and may well penetrate the skull of someone not wearing a helmet; even a stone the size of a small coin falling 50m could do considerable damage. A fall from a rock face that results in bashing your head against the rock could cause severe injury. Still, many climbers don't wear a helmet. It's rare to see climbers at an indoor venue wearing helmets unless they're under supervised instruction. And I don't think I've ever seen a boulderer wearing a helmet – it just wouldn't be cool!

At beginner level you should always wear a helmet both when climbing and when belaying at the base of the crag. When you've gained experience and are a fully-fledged climber in your own right, you're in a much better position to make sound judgements based on personal familiarity and knowledge.

A wide selection of helmets is commercially available. There are those made from a solid polycarbonate shell and those that are variations of the bicycle helmet style of construction. Modern-day helmets are lightweight and available in a range of colour schemes to suit all tastes. Most helmets feature an adjustable internal harness to allow for a perfect fit. A helmet should fit snugly so that, with the chinstrap unsecured, you can nod your head gently back and forth without the helmet falling off.

⬇ **Internal adjustable harnesses vary slightly between manufacturers. A helmet should sit comfortably on your head with the harness adjusted so that it will remain in place when you nod your head but with the chinstrap undone.**

➡ **Light foam-lined helmets are a popular choice.**

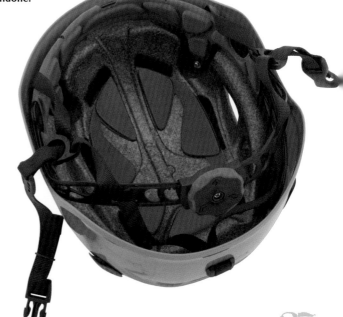

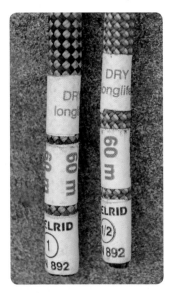

⬆ Various rope diameters, from left: 11mm and 10mm single ropes; 8.5mm and 7.9mm half ropes; 6mm and 5mm accessory cords.

⬅ The UIAA categorisations for single and half rope are clearly marked; the various manufacturers offer clear guidelines for rope storage.

⬇ Ropes can be carried coiled or loosely piled into a bag known as a rope tarp. Placing the rope on a sheet or tarp at the base of a climb will help preserve its longevity and keep it clean. You should avoid standing on a rope at all costs – even small sharp stones can do untold damage.

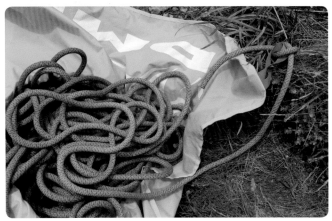

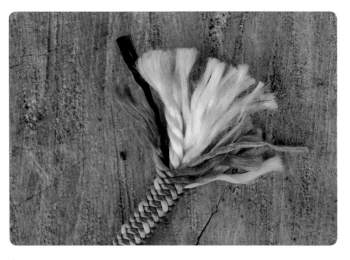

⬆ Climbing ropes are constructed with a core and a sheath, where the bulk of the rope's strength is in the core and the sheath acts mainly as protection. All climbing ropes are made from nylon and the strands that run through them are continuous. Nylon has a fairly low melting point and climbing situations where a moving nylon rope runs over a static rope are to be avoided.

THE ROPE

There's a popular myth that in the old days Joe Brown began climbing with his mother's washing line! Climbing ropes are designed and manufactured specifically for the task. The rope must be strong, hard-wearing and easy to handle. All climbing ropes have the ability to absorb shock gradually, rather like an extremely powerful piece of elastic.

There are two main systems of roped safety in rock climbing. One system uses a single rope and the other uses two ropes that are normally thinner. Rope manufacturers classify ropes for use as single or double; ropes for use in a double-rope system are actually classified as '½ rope'. When you start out, a single-rope system is recommended, and, indeed, for sport climbing and climbing at an indoor wall there's little need for double ropes.

The diameter of the rope is crucial. Single rope diameters range from around 8.9mm to 11mm; this range may not sound particularly wide but the difference in terms of gripping in your hands is significant. The selection you make will very likely depend on budget and the physical weight of the rope. A good compromise is rope around 10mm in diameter, as this is comfortable to grip, fairly light in weight and reasonable cost.

As you gain experience and discover that climbing is what you want to do, you'll almost certainly need to move on to climbing with double ropes, which are normally 8–9mm in diameter. There are advantages to this system when doing long trad climbs that weave around and also if you need to descend a climb by abseil. The use of double ropes is discussed in more detail later in the book.

Ropes come in a variety of lengths. The minimum length to buy is 50m, which will suffice for most climbs. A 60m rope, however, is the preference of most climbers as this gives greater flexibility in choosing the length of pitches that can be tackled both in trad and sport climbing. There are some sport climbs around the world that require much longer ropes, and 70m, 80m and 100m ropes are available if required.

Other diameters of rope are available for purposes other than the main climbing rope. Any rope that's 7mm or less in diameter is usually referred to as accessory cord. The most usual use of 6mm or 7mm cord is to make up Prusik loops (see Chapter 4).

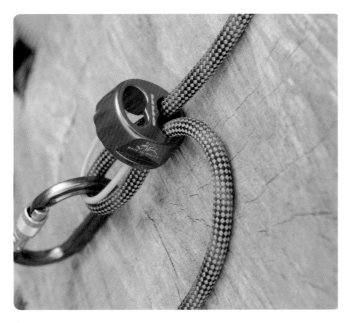

⬆ **A belay device is used to secure the climber's rope and make it easier to hold falls.**

BELAY DEVICE

The rope is the most vital piece of safety equipment for climbers and there are specific devices that climbers use to help them hold the rope securely.

Before the advent of 'mechanical' belay devices, climbers would secure the rope by wrapping it around their waists or over their shoulders. The friction created in using these body-belaying methods helped grip on the rope – but it was very tenuous, uncomfortable and potentially dangerous. If the rope was allowed to run through the hands it would cause horrific burns, to the point where the belayer might actually let go of the rope. This problem would be mitigated if a climber wore gloves and plenty of thickly padded clothing, but in a T-shirt and gloveless on a hot day it could have dire consequences.

This practice was pretty much the only way to hold the rope securely until the early 1970s, when the first belay plate, called a 'Sticht plate', was introduced. Nowadays the plethora of belay devices available makes climbing life much safer.

A belay device works on the basic principle of creating friction through a slotted plate. Bending the unloaded rope over the side of the device can create more friction. The device is attached to the harness using a locking screwgate karabiner with a large rounded curve to it. To operate the device correctly the climber must bear one thing in mind at all times – the unloaded rope must always be securely gripped by at least one hand. We go into more detail about the operation of belay devices in Chapter 5.

Though this type of belay device in all its guises is by far the most common, there are other methods and devices that can be used in slightly different ways, perhaps the most popular of these being the GriGri. For the novice climber, however, the GriGri is rather too specialised and expensive, so it's probably better to save money initially and buy a simpler device.

➡ **When holding the weight of a climber the belayer will lock off the rope as shown; the friction created makes it very secure but you must never let go of the locking or 'controlling' rope.**

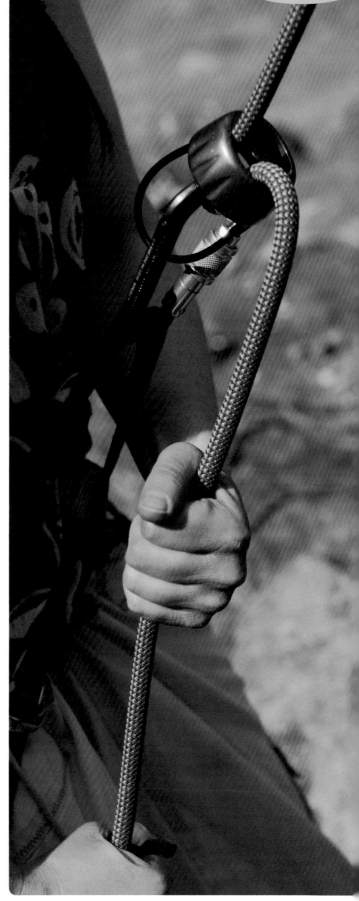

KARABINERS

Most often referred to as 'krabs', these items come in two categories – screwgate and snaplink – and are available in an incredible range of types and sizes.

A screwgate krab is used for attaching the most vital bits of safety gear to the climber's harness or to an anchor point. There are essentially two shapes of screwgate: D-shaped and pear-shaped. The latter is sometimes called HMS, short for 'Halb Mastwurf Sicherung', which translates as 'half securing knot', otherwise known as an Italian hitch. D-shaped krabs, which are the strongest you can buy, are used for general-purpose attachments, whereas pear-shaped krabs are used with belay devices and for securing ropes when you anchor to the rock face.

To lock a screwgate krab, turn the sleeve on the threaded rod until the gate of the krab cannot be opened. There's a design of auto-locking sleeved krab called 'twistlock' that locks up once released; this seems a good idea but in reality requires a knack to operate successfully.

Snaplink krabs are used in situations where the climber needs to deploy them with haste and efficiency. This is usually in a leading situation where the lead climber has to place protection during the ascent. Snaplinks are light, very strong and come with two different choices of gate opening – wire or solid. The advantage of wire is lighter weight; on a climb where you might carry 30 or more snaplinks the weight saving is significant. If you're going to do a good deal of sport climbing, where you'll be clipping into fixed rock anchors, it's a good idea to have sturdy karabiners attached to fairly substantial quickdraws; lightweight wire gates, though perfectly strong, aren't quite as hard-wearing or as easy to grab in an emergency.

CRACK PROTECTION

Crack protection is the collective term for the equipment that forms the basis of all safety for trad climbing. There are two categories of crack protection – nuts and cams.

Nuts range in size from the unbelievably tiny up to large, cowbell-like lumps of alloy. They come in two basic shapes: wedge, of which there are a number of variations, and hex, which feature six angled facets of slightly differing size. Climbers use nuts to make climbing safer by creating anchors to secure themselves to the rock face and to make running belays when leading a climb.

The way in which a nut is placed is simplicity itself: you put it in a

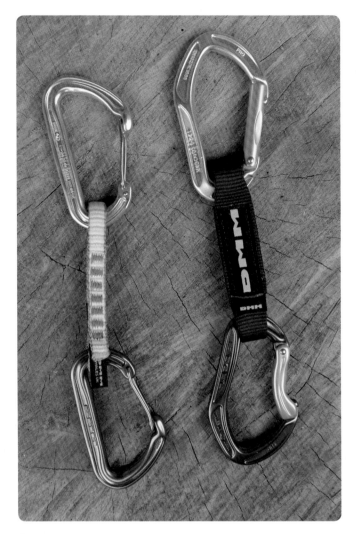

⬆ **There are two types of snaplink karabiner, attached to either end of a quickdraw. Those with wire gates (left) are lighter in weight and those with solid gates (right) are more robust. Of the solid-gate karabiners one has a straight gate and the other a curved gate, which is designed to make clipping in a rope much more efficient.**

⬇ **Screwgate krabs come in a variety of shapes designed for slightly differing purposes. D-shaped karabiners are used for everything except with a belay device. The oval-shaped karabiner is a good 'do-it-all' type of krab while the pear-shaped krab is used mainly for belaying devices and also for securing the rope with clove hitches or Italian hitches.**

⬇ **Pear-shaped or HMS screwgate karabiner with a clove hitch clipped to it.**

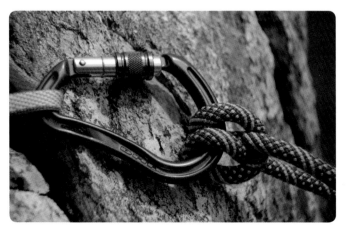

→ **For safety on a climb, you'll need to anchor yourself on ledges part way up and, as shown here, at the top of the climb. There are numerous devices for this purpose.**

crack that tapers and wedge it down until it will go no further, even if a severe load is placed on it. Placing nuts in cracks is an art form and the skill of good placement requires considerable practice. To begin with, it's sensible to practise placing them in a non-critical situation. Find some rock that has a number of crack features where you can stand on the ground and experiment with varying sizes and shapes. In Chapter 5 we take a much more detailed look at how to place nuts.

Most nuts are slung on wire slings swaged or soldered by the manufacturer and rated to a specific strength. It's possible to purchase nuts with a soft nylon sling pre-threaded and stitched by the manufacturer. A mixture of both is ideal.

In the early 1980's American climber Ray Jardine invented a revolutionary device for crack protection. His principle design comprised four cams operating on independent springs. By operating a tigger bar all the cams would close simultaneously and the user could insert the device into a crack. On releasing the trigger bar each cam would open and grip the rock surface. Any downward force would

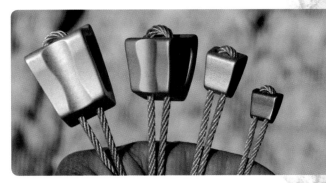

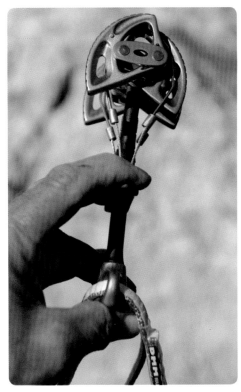

↑ **Wedge-shaped nuts on wire: the aluminium block can be jammed into a crack so that any load forces it tighter into the crack. Various sizes are available, from tiny to huge.**

← **A camming device is a clever gadget used to create a secure anchor in cracks in the rock, particularly those that don't taper in a 'V' shape to suit wedge-shaped nuts.**

force the cams to open even more causing them to bite securely into the rock each side of the crack. The first commercially available cams carried the brand name 'Friends' and to some extent this has become the generic term for similar styles of device.

Cams were a radical step forward at the time and with continuous development by various manufacturers there are now a number of excellent devices that are essential equipment for the rock climber. However, cams are costly, so as a novice you may choose to buy only one or two, gradually building a collection as you gain experience. As with nuts, cams come in a variety of sizes from miniscule to enormous, the latter being weighty and rather specialised pieces of kit.

SLINGS AND QUICKDRAWS

Slings are loops of nylon webbing for placing around spikes or flakes of rock, threading rocks jammed in cracks, wrapping around trees or for extending the attachment to anchors. They can be purchased in a range of standard sizes and the ends are stitched together to form a closed loop. Most modern slings are made from nylon and Dyneema (see panel), which is a high-tensile material that's very hard wearing and adds strength. A useful number and combination of slings is two or three of 2.4m and one or two of 1.2m; sling measurement is by the length of the webbing unstitched.

A quickdraw is a short, sewn sling with a loop at both ends and through these two loops you clip a snaplink karabiner. Quickdraws are used for attaching to bolts fixed into the rock on sport climbs and for adding extensions to crack protection. A sport climbing rack will normally be made up of 10–14 quickdraws and a similar number is adequate for trad climbing, though climbers often carry quickdraws in a number of varying lengths.

CHALK BAG

Chalk or magnesium carbonate is used to increase grip on handholds. When hands become sweaty it's more difficult to grip the rock. This is most noticeable when the climber tries to use tiny finger holds and particularly when the combination of hot weather and an element of fear are prevalent. At lower grades of difficulty this is rarely a problem and the use of chalk is hardly necessary, but on more difficult and technical rock climbs, as well as indoor climbing and bouldering, chalk is pretty much essential.

A chalk bag is usually quite small – you should be able to get one hand comfortably into it to chalk up the fingertips. Chalk comes in two forms: block chalk, which is crumbled into the bag, and powdered chalk, which is encased in a muslin ball. Chalk balls are the only form permitted at indoor climbing venues; block chalk tends to be less fine and sticks to the fingers better.

Climbers first used chalk in the late 1970s and it caused a huge outcry among some in the climbing fraternity. Some climbers said that it was cheating and, more significantly, left an ugly mark on the rock. The debate has largely subsided nowadays but there are still a few climbers for whom the use of chalk is anathema.

BOULDERING MAT

Many bouldering sites have hazardous ground below and during attempts to solve a boulder problem you may well fall off awkwardly. As well as having mates to look after you so that you don't land on your back or otherwise injure yourself, it's also essential to use a bouldering mat to help create a soft landing place. If everyone in a group of boulderers brings along a mat, you can build up a fairly comfortable landing zone – but don't expect it to be as soft as a feather mattress!

WHAT IS DYNEEMA?

Dyneema and nylon are synthetic raw materials used in the construction of slings and quickdraws for climbing. Dyneema is a polyethylene whereas nylon is a polyamide. Dyneema has a much greater strength-to-weight ratio than nylon, it's more resistant to abrasion and less susceptible to UV degradation, and it doesn't absorb water. However, it has much less elasticity than nylon and is therefore less dynamic when it comes to absorbing impact loads. It also has a much lower melting point than nylon.

Dyneema is usually mixed with a proportion of nylon to achieve ideal handling properties for rock climbing applications. This 'best of both worlds' blend provides the climber with lightweight, high-strength safety equipment. Spectra is another brand of very similar material.

⬇ **Slings are an essential part of climbing safety. Made of nylon interlaced with Dyneema, they're used to create anchors around flakes of rock and rocks jammed in cracks, called chockstones, and also to create safe multiple-anchor points.**

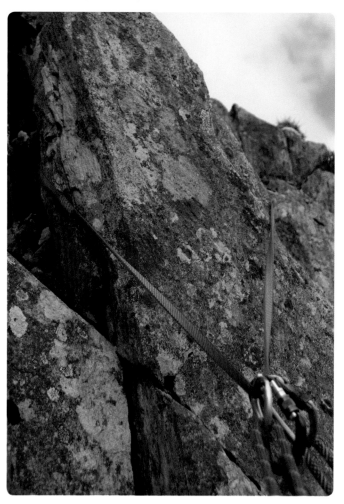

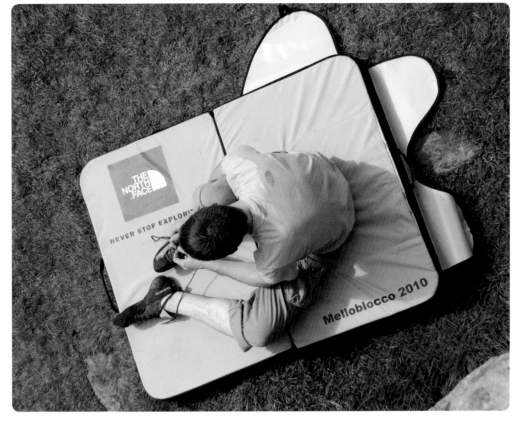

← Placed at the base of a boulder to soften a landing, bouldering mats have become essential equipment during the rise of bouldering as a sport in its own right.

↓ A now-familiar sight in the outdoors – the strange profile of the boulderer!

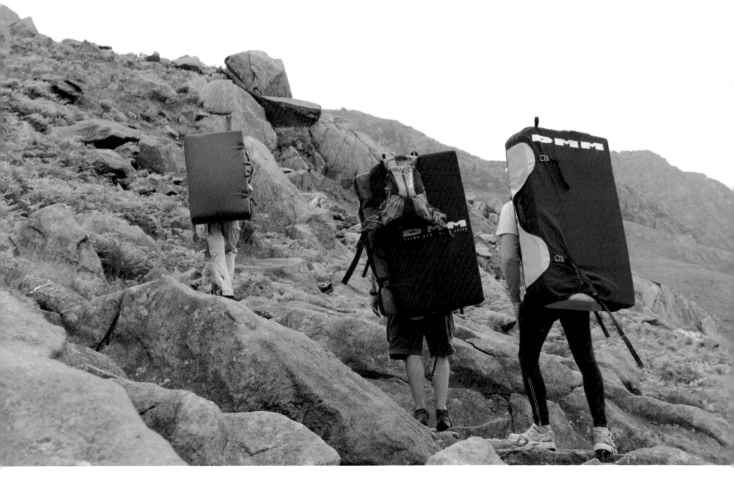

NUT KEY

This is an essential tool that each climber carries. Sometimes called a 'furkler' by older climbers, a nut key is used to help release nuts and cams that become impossible to reach with the fingers or so tightly stuck that fingers alone won't loosen them. There's a variety of makes and designs, all of which look similar and work well.

GUIDEBOOKS

Information about how to find crags and cliffs and the routes to climb is widely available in climbing guidebooks.

There's a long tradition of guidebook writing, particularly in the UK, where the style of description is often couched in terms completely alien to the non-climber. This jargon takes time to learn, as does the interpretation of guidebook nomenclature. For example, a climb that is described as 'interesting' will almost certainly have some kind of unexpected and nasty twist. A climb described as 'bold' will probably lack adequate and comforting protection for the leader. 'Delicate' is likely to mean a climb that is devoid of reassuring handholds and footholds.

Alongside the description of the climb there will be a grade, as shown in the accompanying table. Grading standards vary from country to country; useful comparisons can be made within one country's grading system, but otherwise this is an area that's always open to criticism and debate.

In the UK there's a two-tier grading system. The adjectival grade is an overall interpretation of the level of seriousness of the undertaking. From this you can see that the grade 'Diff' (Difficult) is considerably less serious than the highest grade of 'E10'. Climbs of 'Diff' grade aren't usually particularly steep and are generally blessed with large handholds and footholds, and lots of ledges on which to take a break. Climbs at

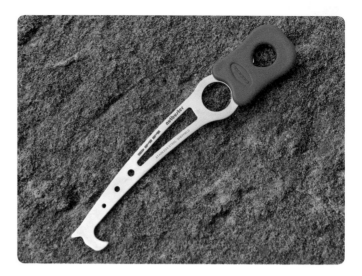

⬆ **A nut key or 'furkler' is an essential tool to help extract a nut or cam stuck in a crack.**

'E10' are undertaken only rarely and by those who have 'special powers' of ability and strength, as well as an extremely cool head. The middle ground of grades from 'VS' through to 'E4' is where most climbers operate and where you'll find some of the most satisfying climbs.

To a certain extent the adjectival grade will also tell you how difficult the moves on a climb will be – but not entirely. To help make the distinction between overall grade and technical difficulty, climbers use a grading system adapted from one used in Europe. The technical

CLIMBING GRADES: INTERNATIONAL COMPARISONS

UK (adjective)	UK (technical)	UIAA	French (sport)	USA	Australia
Moderate (M or Mod)	N/A	I to II	I	5.1–5.2	4–5
Difficult (D or Diff)	N/A	II to III+	I to 2+	5.2–5.3	5–7
Very Difficult (VD or V Diff)	N/A	III to III+	2 to 3-	5.2–5.4	6–8
Hard Very Difficult (HVD or Hard V Diff)	N/A	III+ to IV+	2+ to 3-	5.4–5.6	8–10
Mild Severe (MS)	N/A	IV to IV+	3- to 3+	5.5–5.6	10–11
Severe (S)	4a–4b	IV to V-	3 to 4	5.5–5.7	10–12
Hard Severe (HS)	4a–4c	IV+ to V	3 to 4+	5.6–5.7	12–13
Mild Very Severe (MVS)	4a–4c	IV+ to V	3+ to 4+	5.6–5.7	12–14
Very Severe (VS)	4a–4c	V- to V+	4 to 5	5.7–5.8	13–15
Hard Very Severe (HVS)	4c–5b	V+ to VI	4+ to 6a	5.8–5.9	15–18
E1	5a–5c	VI to VI+	5+ to 6a+	5.9–5.10a	18–20
E2	5b–6a	VI+ to VII	6a+ to 6b+	5.10b–5.10c	19–21
E3	5c–6a	VII to VII+	6b to 6c	5.10d–5.11b	20–22
E4	6a–6b	VII+ to VIII	6c to 7a	5.11b–5.11d	22–23
E5	6a–6c	VIII to IX-	7a to 7b	5.11d–5.12b	23–25
E6	6b–6c	IX- to IX+	7b to 7c+	5.12b–5.13a	25–28
E7	6c–7a	IX+ to X	7c+ to 8a+	5.13a–5.13c	28–30
E8	6c–7a	X to X+	8a+ to 8b+	5.13c–5.14a	30–32
E9	7a–7b	X+ to XI	8b+ to 8c+	5.14a–5.14c	32–34
E10	7a–7b	XI to XI+	8c+ to 9a+	5.14c–5.15a	34–36

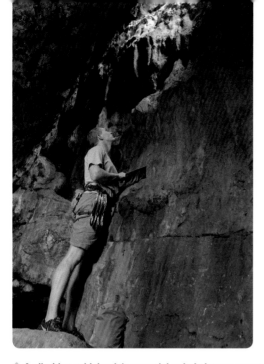

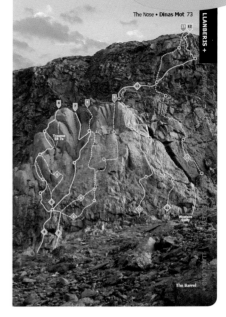

↑ A climbing guidebook is essential to help locate crags to climb and routes up those crags. Even with a guidebook, actually locating a climb can sometimes be tricky, and interpreting what is stated about a particular climb can be challenging because the language is often couched in somewhat devious terms.

↑ The layouts and descriptions in guidebooks vary from detailed and flowery at one extreme to a simple photo or diagram (often called a 'topo') with the line of the route marked on it, together with the route name and a grade.

grade will only give the climber an idea of how difficult a sequence of moves on each climb or pitch will be. The system doesn't usually kick in until the 'Very Severe' grade. At this point it begins with 4a, 4b and 4c, and then goes up in numbered increments using the same letters right up to 8a, 8b and 8c; thus we have 15 grades of technical difficulty.

The UK grading system is further complicated by the fact that the system used to grade sport climbs (those protected by fixed bolts) is the same as that used in France and other European countries; indeed, it's sometimes referred to as the 'French' grade. As a very rough comparison, a 5a grade for a trad climb would equate to a 4b sport grade. This two-grade difference can be applied across all the technical grades in order to make vague comparisons!

Knowing the grade of a climb is essential when choosing a route, to be sure that you don't take on a challenge that's way beyond your ability and experience.

The climbers who make the first ascent of a climb are entitled to give the climb a name. The variety of route names is as diverse as you might imagine. Long ago climbs were usually named after a feature on a crag or cliff, so you might have Arête Climb or Crack Climb. Nowadays all sorts of connotations are used and climb names may follow a specific theme on one crag or may be seemingly named at random. Usually there's a specific reason why a climb has a particular name and often it's known only to those who pioneered the climb.

There's a considerable amount of work undertaken to keep guidebooks fresh and up to date. A growing trend in such publications is to dispense with the detailed description and show a photograph or artistic drawing of the crag or cliff and to mark a line where each different route goes. These routes will be given a number that corresponds to brief information on the page stating the name of the climb and its grade, and sometimes a few words about the climb. This type of guidebook is particularly useful at sport climbing venues where climbs may be short and numerous.

There are so many climbing areas around the world, some quite small, that not all climbing crags are featured in any guidebook. Information is available online, of course, and some guidebook publishers offer downloadable mini-guides for purchase.

Most guidebook writers also use a star-rating system for the quality of the overall experience. A three-star climb will have all the attributes necessary for a thoroughly enjoyable climbing experience, such as the situation, the quality of the rock and the perceived adventure aspect. Needless to say 'starred' climbs are always the most frequented and on a sunny weekend you'll have to arrive early if you want to be the first on the climb.

↓ Guidebooks are a source of great inspiration to climbers and building up a library can be very expensive, but, as someone once remarked, the more climbs you do from a particular guidebook the better value it becomes…

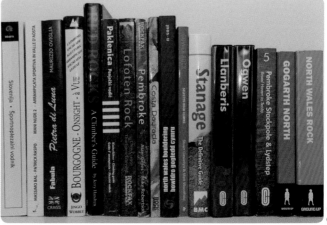

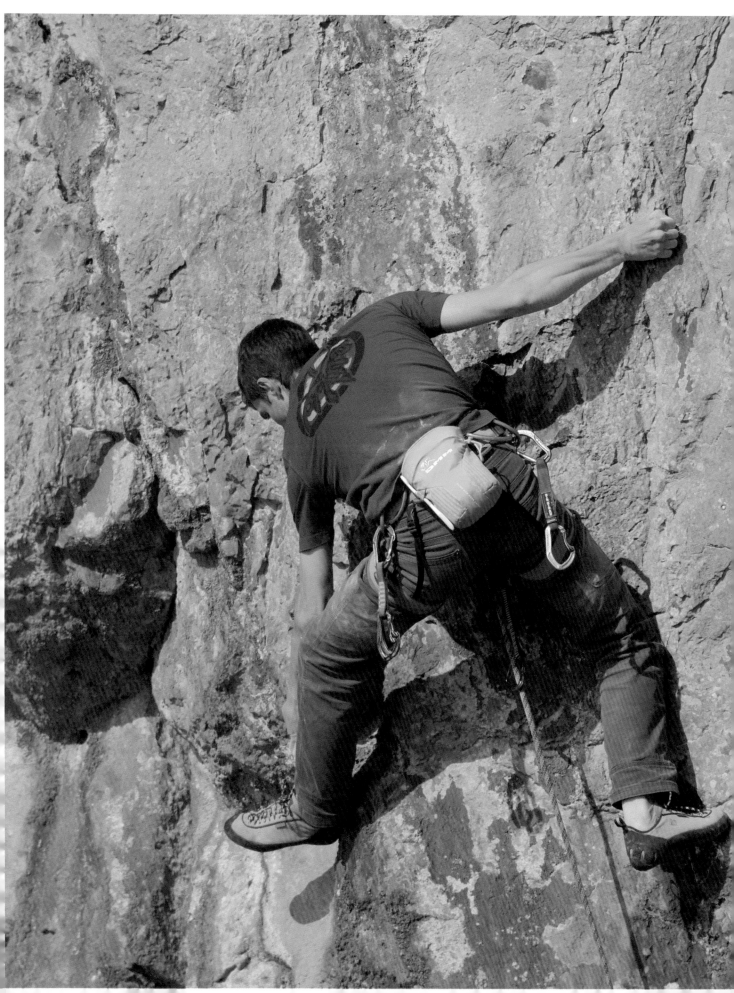

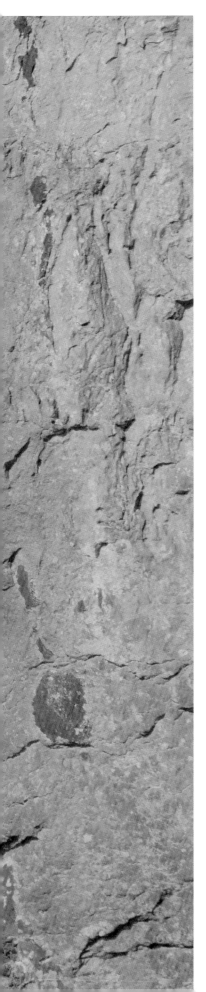

CHAPTER 3

CLIMBING TECHNIQUE

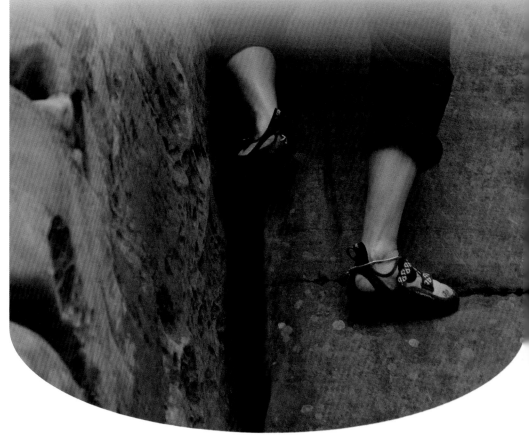

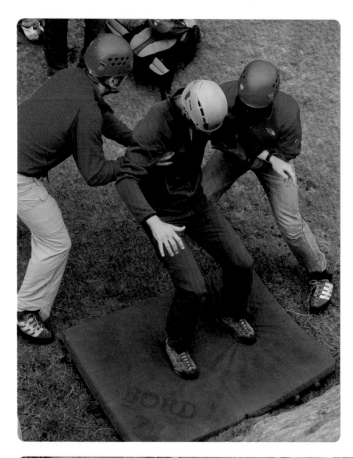

If you're blessed with strength, agility, a cool head and confidence in your own physical ability, you're a true descendant of the ape and can skip this chapter and go climbing immediately! If not, you're among the remaining 99 per cent of the climbing population and will almost certainly benefit from a few points of guidance.

The first experiences of rock climbing are vital to the long-term enjoyment and pleasures that are possible. However, a traumatic experience early on can put off a novice forever, and over the years I've met many people who described their first experience of rock climbing as the most terrifying thing they'd ever done and had no intention of trying it again. But I've also met many more people who had a similar first experience but went on to become fully committed rock climbers.

The first steps are very important and need to be taken in as comfortable an environment as possible. Aspirations and expectations may be high but initially need to be tempered with common sense.

← **Practise climbing techniques with a group of like-minded people. Indoors or outdoors you need to buddy up and look after each other. It isn't about catching them if they fall but more about ensuring they don't fall awkwardly.**

↓ **Be ready to help at any time and be reassuring.**

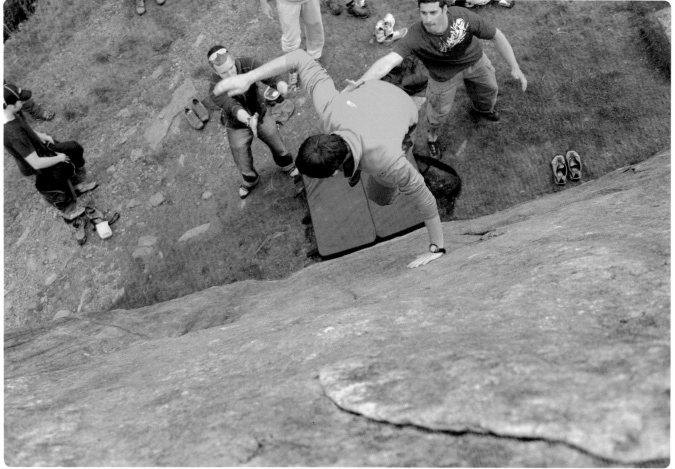

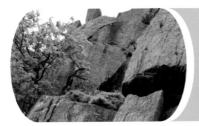

WHERE TO BEGIN

For many, the first experience of climbing will be at an indoor climbing wall. This is a very good place to start, particularly as weather won't affect you. Indoors there will be climbs set up specifically for beginners, with low angles and featuring large, plentiful holds for both feet and hands. Not all venues, however, will offer the full gamut of possible types and styles of movement.

Outdoors you'll have to be a little more careful about where to begin. The worst introduction would be on wet, slippery rock. An ideal venue would feature lots of low-angled rough rock (slabs), not too high above the ground, with lush, grassy meadows below. To progress, the ideal next step would be a smattering of steeper rock with features such as vertical and horizontal cracks, and maybe one or two wider cracks that you can get into with part or all of your body.

CLIMBING NOMENCLATURE

BLOCK This could be free-standing, wedged or jammed. Usually it's at least body-sized but it could be the size of a large car.

FLAKE A detached piece of rock that may or may not be wedged or jammed in place. It could also be quite a tiny feature as part of the rock face.

CRACK Anything from a few millimetres wide to something that you can't quite get your body into.

CHIMNEY A large crack that you can easily get your body into.

CORNER Rather like an open book, square-cut corners can be very pronounced (with large walls either side) or less obvious.

GROOVE A shallow corner rather like a book opened out on a table; this is not at all square-cut and may be nothing more than a shallow runnel.

OVERHANG A piece of jutting-out rock that can be reached around.

ROOF A very large overhang, the sort of edifice that would provide shelter in a storm or even a space that could be lived in.

OVERLAP A very small overhang.

SLAB A relatively smooth slab of rock at an angle of 30–60 degrees.

WALL A more vertical slab of rock; if the angle exceeds 90 degrees it's called an overhanging wall.

LEDGE Simply a ledge…

ARÊTE A feature that sticks out prominently from the rest of the face or from the edge of a rock face. The angle between the two sides can be quite narrow or quite wide. If the edge is round, the feature is called a rounded arête. The American term 'outside corner' is perhaps more descriptive.

CRAG AND ROCK FEATURES

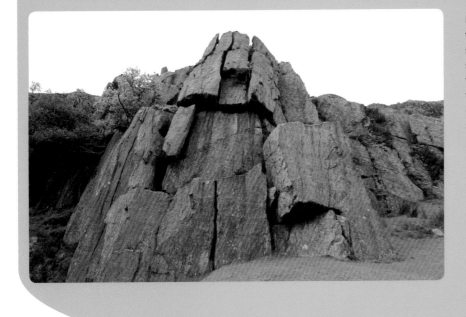

It's rare that a rock face is smooth and featureless. Huge expanses of granite slabs or walls may appear unvarying and smooth but there will usually be fine features that can be identified only from close up. Normally all kinds of cracks, overhangs, overlaps, corners and grooves, to name but a few, feature on crags.

This photo illustrates a number of crag features and the nomenclature that's in common use among rock climbers. Understanding these features will help the climber to anticipate what techniques may be required for a successful ascent, though having a particular expectation may be proved worthless on closer inspection.

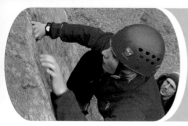

THE BASICS OF MOVEMENT

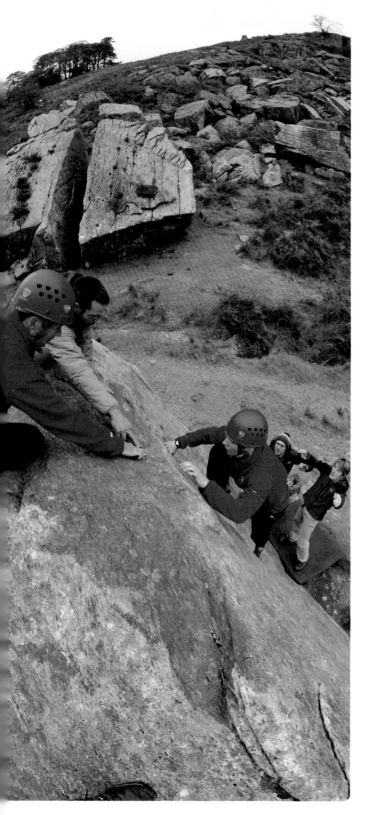

It's all about footwork! Contrary to the commonly held belief that all climbers need to be as strong as monkeys, excellent footwork is the key to good technique.

As stated in the previous section, it's really important to choose a suitable venue, whether indoors or outdoors, to practise climbing techniques. Ideally it's better to remain close to the ground so that if you slip off you can comfortably jump to the ground without hurting yourself. It's sensible to practise moves with companions in attendance who remain vigilant to your every move and can help you land properly should you slip off. This is called 'spotting' or 'buddying up'. Buddies aren't there to catch you in their arms if you slip but rather to ensure that you don't topple backwards when you land. They can also be useful in offering a reassuring hand on your back to help you maintain balance while you make moves.

To begin with experiment a little with what your climbing shoes can do, and again a low-angled slab is perfect for this. Try a little exercise where you use only your fingertips for balance and tiptoe around on the rock carefully 'smearing' all of the front sole against the rock surface. This should give you confidence in the way the rubber can 'stick' to the rock. If you get worried you can always use your hands to grip the available handholds.

Don't just climb in an upward direction, but try to move sideways and downwards too. The key thing here is to take only tiny steps. Don't try to get your foot up by your ear just yet.

Gradually move on to slightly steeper rock until you find that it becomes less easy to get a grip with the soles of the shoes by just 'smearing' them over the surface. At this point begin to search the rock for little edges, shallow scoops or small irregularities that might provide a more secure grip. Surprisingly, these need not be huge foot ledges but might be tiny hollows or thin, flat edges on which you can stand.

Using the shoes across the width of the sole and standing on the inside or outside rim of the shoe will provide greater and more secure support than attempting to stand directly over the front of the toe.

As you move over the rock, keep looking down at where the next foothold might be and plan an efficient series of foot movements to reach the holds you spot.

An old-fashioned saying, often bandied about, states that you should always maintain three points of contact with the rock, and that you should never lean in, cross your feet or use your knees. However, you should ignore most of this and do what comes most naturally, though the point about not using your knees is sound advice.

Once you get bored with padding around, move on to a similar exercise but on steeper rock where you have to use handholds. These may not necessarily be huge 'rung-of-a-ladder' holds, but something over which you can curl the top two joints of your fingers will be sufficient for a secure grip.

Climbers use the term 'positive' hold for handholds and footholds that present a clean and obvious edge on which to hold or stand. 'Positive' holds are just what you need when starting out.

← **Having someone to point out crucial holds is extremely helpful.**

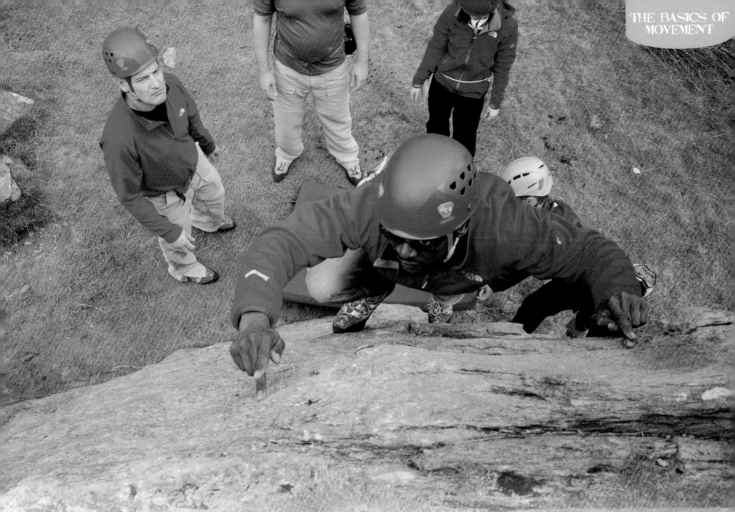

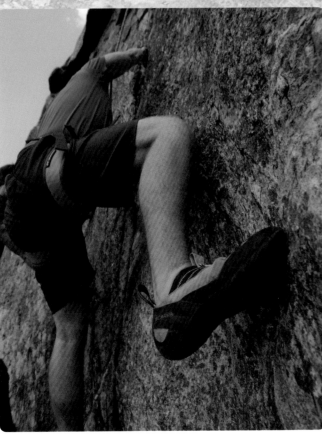

Building trust and confidence in your footwork is vital to efficient climbing. You cannot climb on brawn alone.

Even the tiniest of scoops or corrugations can provide good grip for the feet.

A pronounced edge is an obvious foothold.

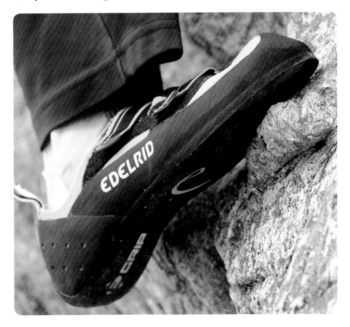

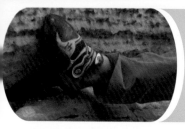

TYPES OF FOOTHOLD

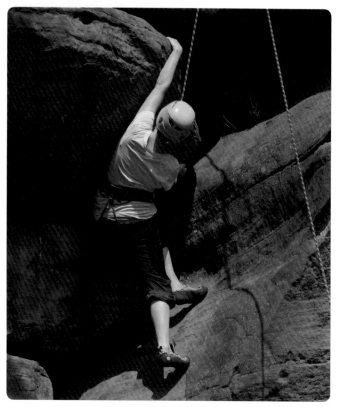

SMEARING

This is a friction foothold where you rely mainly on sole-to-rock contact. Smearing is only effective as long as you keep weight over the sole; any unweighting releases the friction and your foot will probably slip off the rock. Smearing advantages can be gained by grinding the sole into the tiny ripples and crystals in the rock face. As such, some rock types – such as granite and gritstone – lend themselves better to smearing than others. Slate and limestone, which are often polished by the passage of thousands of feet, aren't so good.

← Where there are no obvious ledges or edges for footholds, the sticky nature of the rubber sole of a rock shoe enables the climber to 'smear' the sole over the rock. Provided that body weight is kept over the foot and the heel dropped low, the foot should remain in place and give an excellent and comfortable foothold.

⬇ A very smooth slab: the climber is totally reliant on friction and needs to be confident that feet will stick to the rock. The handholds are large and confidence inspiring, allowing the climber to experiment with the amount of pressure required to aid upward movement.

⬇ Very rough rock such as granite has excellent friction properties, enabling the climber to have great confidence in a smeared foothold. Here tiny barnacles below the high-tide mark offer friction on the rock face; the rock is limestone.

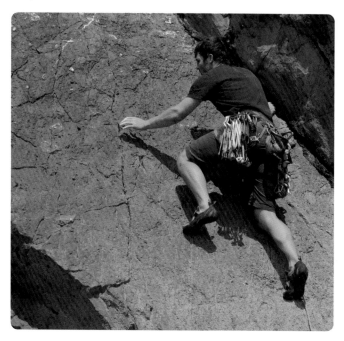

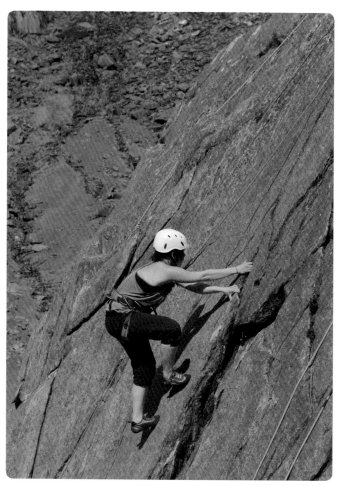

EDGING

Edging is where the inside or outside rim of the climbing shoe sole is placed on an edge of rock. Edges, which range from only 1–2mm up to 1cm, can be sharp and well defined or slightly sloping.

The smaller the edge, the greater the confidence required. When you practise this technique, first try it close to the ground. A combination of edging and smearing is sometimes possible on lower-angled rock.

FOOT JAMMING

Foot jamming is used in cracks where no obvious edges or smears can be used. The most comfortable foot jams are where a crack is as wide as the foot and tapers slightly, allowing the foot to be wedged into the crack. The most uncomfortable foot jams are where the crack is slightly narrower than the width of the foot and the shoe must be placed in the crack sideways and then twisted to secure it in place.

Cracks that need to be climbed entirely using foot jams are very tiring and tough on the feet, so only do short sections to begin with.

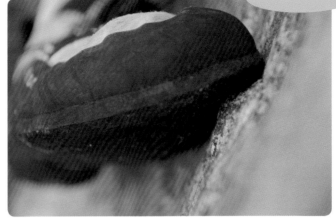

⬆ **If edges, no matter how small, present themselves, you can stand on the inside toe of the rock shoe; the foot needs to be turned so the heel points slightly inward.**

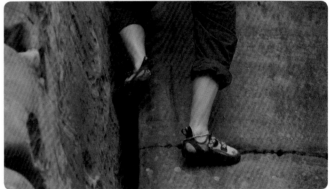

⬆ **It's possible to wedge the feet into cracks in the rock. The simplest is to simply place it in a crack that's a similar width to your foot and move it into a position where it becomes stuck, then stand up on it. Here the right foot is turned sideways to take advantage of an edge.**

⬅ **Where the crack is narrower than the width of the foot, insert the foot sideways and then twist it until it grips into the crack. In extremely narrow cracks you may only just be able to get the tip of your toe in – but the technique and principle are the same.**

⬇ **This crack is too wide for a sideways foot jam so the foot is wedged lengthways across the crack. It's rather less secure than the previous foot jams, and rather more painful.**

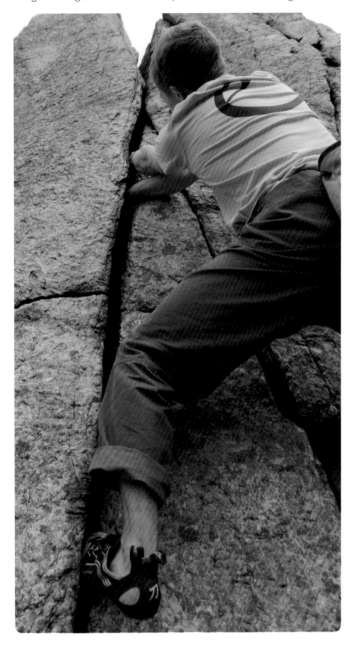

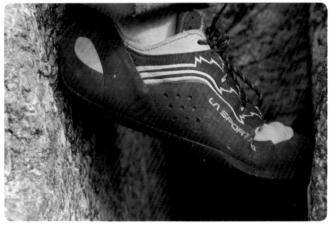

A jug handhold instils enormous confidence and when you have two side by side anything is possible. Here the left hand is on a sharp-edged jug and the right on something a little more rounded but equally reassuring.

Like all climbing sequences, when and how you reach and use handholds is often dependent on your height. But rest assured – some of the very finest climbers aren't tall!

JUG

The jug or jug handle is the most reassuring and biggest type of handhold. You can curl your whole hand over a jug and this will give you enormous confidence to hang off it and pull your body weight up the rock face. Two jugs side by side, sometimes known as 'bucket' holds or 'Thank God' holds, provide bombproof security – so much so that you may be loath to let go of them.

The next best handhold is one over which you can curl the top two joints of the fingers. This type of hold is nearly as comforting as a jug but it does require a little more finger strength and tenacity if you're on steep rock. On lower-angled rock it will give a secure handhold when combined with your feet taking some of the weight.

➜ **A strong handhold using just the fingers curled over an edge is the next best thing to a jug. Here the thumb is also used to grip a protruding edge, further enhancing the overall grip.**

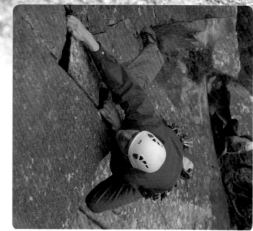

After making a sequence of moves with small handholds, the 'Thank God' holds of jugs offer comfort.

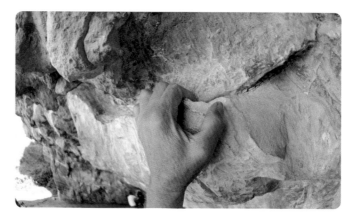

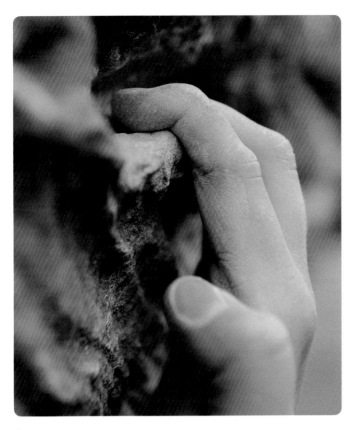

↑ **An open-handed finger hold, using the top joint of the finger.**

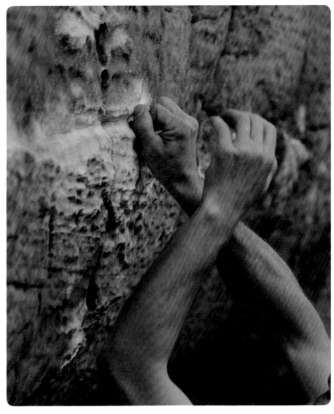

↑ **A crimped finger hold, using mainly the tips of the fingers and supported by the thumb.**

FINGER HOLD

Decreasing in size, the finger hold is where you curl or place only the top joint of the fingers over the hold; usually a finger hold will exclude the little finger.

CRIMP

Next down is the type of hold usually called a crimp, where you can only rest your fingertips on an edge. This may be a flat edge on the rock face or little more than a ripple. If it's particularly tiny, you may only be able to get two fingertips on it.

POCKET

Some types of rock, limestone particularly, feature small holes known as pockets. Some pockets are large enough to be classed as jugs, but others are much smaller and you may only be able to insert one or two fingers; a one-finger pocket is called a 'mono doigt'. Obviously holds of this type require extremely good technique along with a higher degree of finger strength.

JAMS

It's possible to gain a secure handhold in a seemingly smooth-sided crack by using hand-jamming techniques. There are three main types of hold and all are very effective if done correctly, but they're also fairly painful. However, it's rare to need to use jams on easier climbs so at

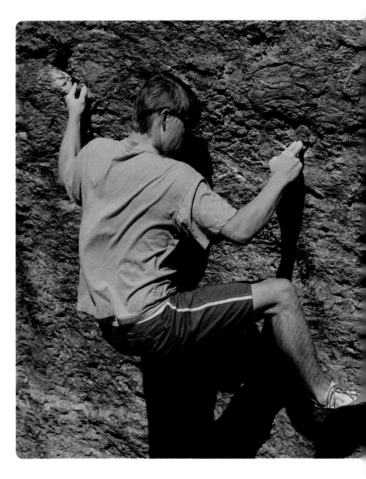

➡ **A two-finger pocket – rather extreme at beginner level but on lower-angled rock with excellent footholds it might be used to help maintain balance.**

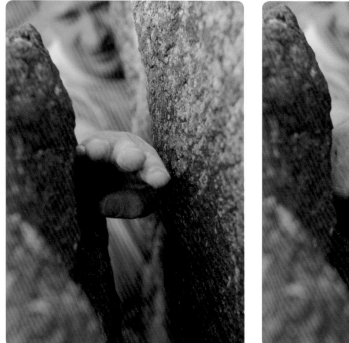

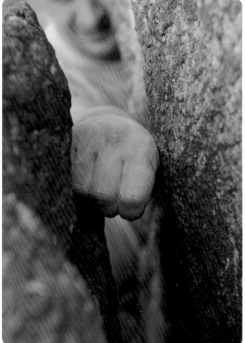

← **When a crack is too wide for a hand jam, you can use a fist. Push your thumb into the palm of your hand and tighten the fist so the skin stretches tight. Wriggle your fist around until it feels secure and tight in the crack.**

least for a while you can be spared the agonising torture! For climbs that feature extreme and prolonged jamming, climbers use tape to protect the skin.

Fist jam

This is used in a crack that's very slightly narrower than the size of your clenched fist. The hand is placed in the crack and the fingers clenched to form a tight fist. The thumb can be placed inside the palm of the hand and gripped tightly to stretch the skin over the back of the hand. This reduces the possibility of tearing the skin.

Hand jam

The hand jam is used in a crack that's slightly narrower than fist width. A well-placed hand jam is as good as a jug – though it may not feel like it at first. The hand is placed inside the crack with fingers on one side and the back of the hand against the opposite side. Push the thumb into the palm of your hand and bend the fingers at the knuckle to create a wedge shape. Tighten the hand into the crack by taking your weight on it.

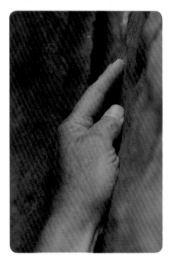

← **A handjam – insert the open hand into the crack…**

→ **… and push the thumb into the palm of your hand. Arch your hand so that the fingers push against one side of the crack with the back of the hand against the other. Wriggle it around until it seats well and try to keep the skin stretched by creating more of an arch across the crack.**

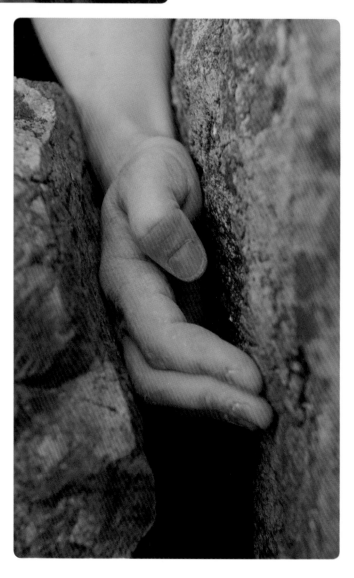

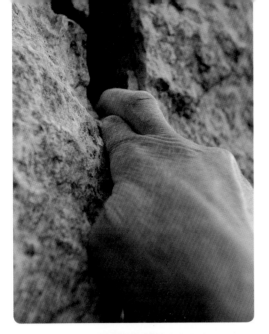

← A rather unusual finger lock, where the ring finger is placed over the forefinger to create a wider profile.

Finger jam

The finger jam is used in even narrower cracks. How you use a finger jam depends on the shape and width of the crack. Ideally you'll be able to get all four fingers in the crack. The hand is then twisted at the wrist to force the fingers to twist inside the crack and tighten on the sides. A variation of this is to place two fingers in the crack, the middle and forefinger, and create a jam where the middle finger is placed over the top of the forefinger; the fingers are then seated in the crack by a twisting action.

FLAT HANDHOLD

A flat handhold, or 'flatty', is one where there isn't so much of an edge to grip on to but all of the fingers can be seated over the hold and the hand bent at the knuckles as far as is possible. The best position to pull up on a flat handhold is normally from directly underneath. As you gain height on the hold it becomes much less effective.

ROUNDED HANDHOLD

A rounded handhold is one where you're able to grip in an open-handed style. If the hold is slightly bulbous, it'll provide a better grip that relies mainly on the friction of the hand over the rock.

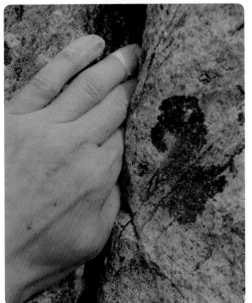

← A finger lock can be very painful but extremely secure. Here's a way to simply jam your fingers as deeply as possible into a tapering crack. By creating a slight twist on the hand the jam is secured.

⬇ A rounded, open-grip handhold may not seem particularly friendly, but sometimes it's all that's available and so you must rely mainly on good footwork to take much of your body weight.

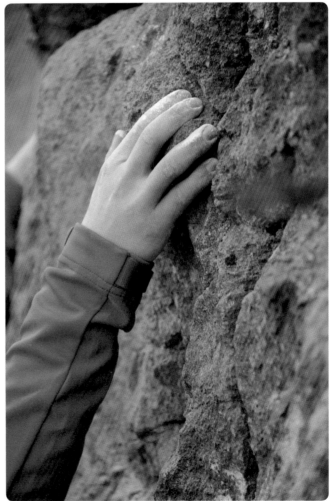

⬇ A flat handhold but with a pronounced edge is good as long as your weight remains directly below. As you move your weight upwards, a flat handhold quickly becomes much less effective.

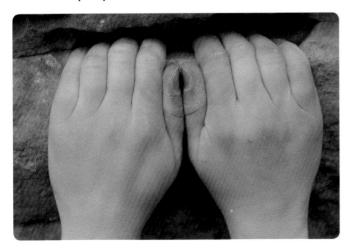

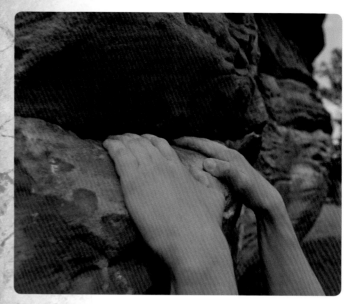

A sloping ledge is another type of tenuous handhold. Like a flat handhold, a sloping ledge is often good when you're directly below but rapidly lose its effectiveness as you gain height.

A sloping finger hold is hardly anything to hang on to. By trusting your feet and pushing up on powerful leg muscles it might just be enough to reach the sharp edge that's coming up next.

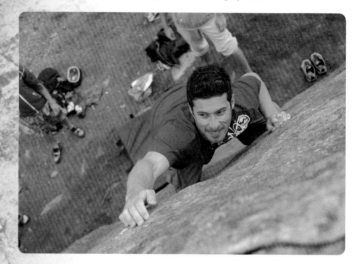

SLOPER

This is exactly what it sounds like – nothing very much to grip on to or curl fingers around, but enough friction can be generated to keep the hand in place.

PINCH GRIP

A pinch grip is again self-explanatory: a piece of rock is gripped between the fingers and thumb. On more difficult climbs there may be pinch grips that can be used by only one finger and the thumb.

The left hand is holding a pinch grip. Quite often you'll be able to curl the fingers over something while the thumb needs only to squeeze against the rock. Like many handholds, on steep rock you'll need more power to use it than you might on lower-angled rock where feet and legs can take much of the strain.

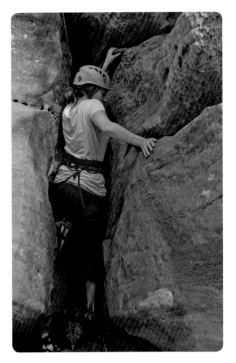

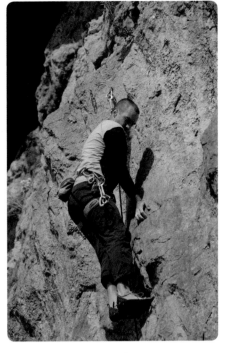

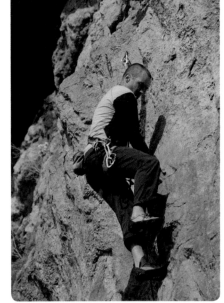

⬆ **Palming is when you push down flat on the rock handhold. It's often used in conjunction with a sound handhold for the other hand and helps you to reposition your body weight over your feet.**

PALMING

Palming is a pressure handhold that can be used on a flat rock surface where the climber relies on friction to keep the hand in place or where there may be an edge or hollow to push against. Palming can be used two ways: in a downward pushing manner or sideways to help maintain balance.

LAYAWAY

A sideways handhold is often called a layaway. This may be the size of a jug or in extreme cases a tiny edge of rock just big enough for a couple of fingers, and the shape may be rounded or even sloping. These types of handhold are most useful if you need to lean across the rock to reach for another handhold or to pull yourself across the rock face.

⬇ **A layaway is used to hold the body in balance while reaching sideways for another handhold. It might also be used as a side pull to help maintain the body in a resting position on the rock.**

⬆ ⬈ **Here the climber has a good handhold with the left hand and can confidently push down on the right hand, enabling him to lift the right foot to make a fairly high step.**

⬇ **Two very fierce side holds. The left is on a very sloping hold while the right is held in more of a crimp style. The next handhold will be one finger in each pocket or hole above with the left hand, and then the right will reach up for the rounded edge directly above. Yes... it's as difficult as it looks.**

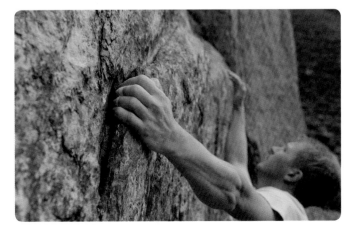

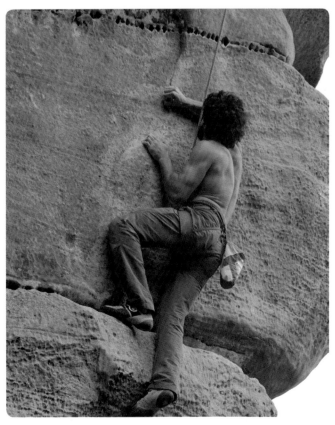

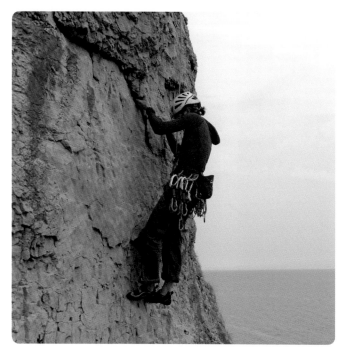

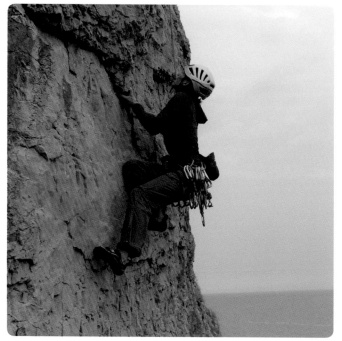

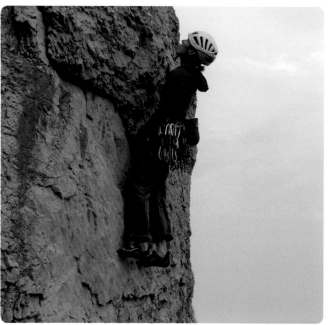

The undercut, or undercling, is a very useful hold if the opportunity ever presents itself. From below, the edge is held in a pinch-type grip while the feet are moved higher. As the feet come up the grip can be changed to pull outwards and slightly upwards, helping you to maintain balance and also to reach higher and further with the other hand for what might be a good handhold.

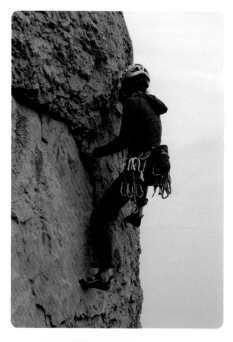

UNDERCUT

An undercut, or undercling, can be a very useful hold, particularly on steeper rock where it can be used to hold your body close to the rock and allow you to keep most of your weight over your feet. This type of hold is also extremely handy in allowing you to make a long reach upwards with the other hand, particularly when reaching around obstacles such as overhangs or overlaps in the rock face.

SLAPPER

A slapper is where you see a handhold up above and make a lunge for it, slapping your hand on to it!

→ **An undercut pinch grip is a combo hold for use in extreme situations.**

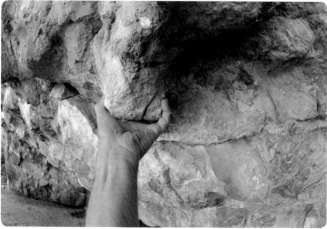

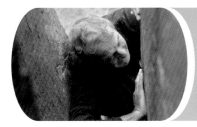

CLIMBING MOVES

This section explains the various moves you're likely to need as you develop your climbing skills and attempt more challenging routes.

MANTLESHELF

In its most simplistic form, a mantleshelf is a technique used to reach a flat ledge where there are no available handholds above the ledge. It's a very dynamic technique that requires a certain degree of strength and suppleness, and a determination not to use a knee! Always explore other ways to get on to a ledge, but if none exists make sure you do the mantleshelf as one fairly fluid movement, using any momentum to make the final step up on to the ledge.

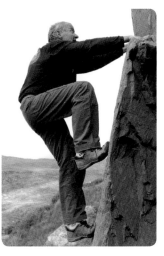

⬆ **A mantleshelf is another dynamic and fairly energetic sequence of moves. Hands are placed on the edge of the ledge and the feet are run up as high as possible.**

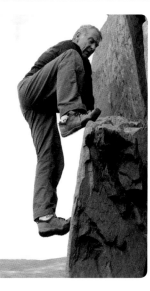

⬆ **Convert the hand-holds into two pressure or palming holds on the edge of the ledge.**

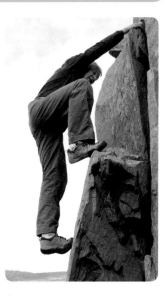

⬆ **Using a fairly fluid motion bring first one foot and then the other up on to ledge as you straighten your arms and then use powerful leg muscles to stand upright. If handholds are available above use them!**

LAYBACKING

A linked series of moves utilising only layaway holds in the same direction is called a layback. The feet are essential in laybacking and create an opposing force to the hands, enabling upward progress. It requires a

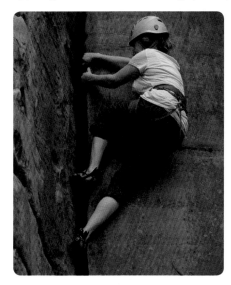

⬆ **Laybacking is a powerful technique where the hands and feet work in opposition to each other. Here the holds are good and the angle not too steep. The initial foothold for the right foot is a foot jam, the climber lays back on her hands and pushes against the opposite wall with her left foot.**

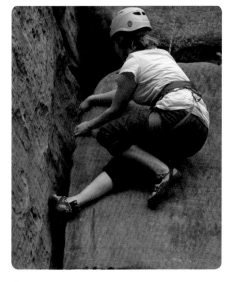

⬆ **The layback position is maintained but here the left foot is placed on a tiny scoop using the outside of the foot. This will take some weight, relieving pressure on the arms.**

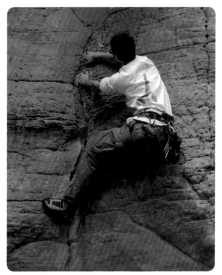

⬆ **Extreme laybacking, using tiny finger holds and much less secure foot placements. The principles remain the same but here it'll be a couple of layback moves only.**

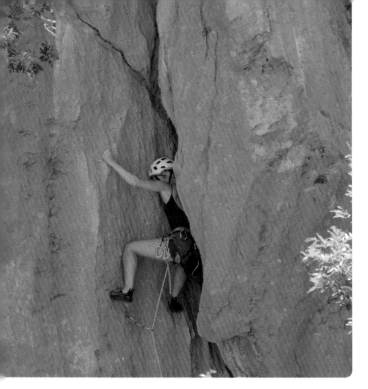

good deal of commitment and prolonged sequences of laybacking are extremely strenuous. It's often difficult to stop once you embark on a layback but if there are small ledges for the feet it might be possible to gain a rest.

CHIMNEYING

A chimney is a crack in the rock face that you can get into with your whole body. Chimneys can be climbed using the back and hands against one side and the feet flat on the other, a technique that's also called 'back and footing'.

Variations to the technique can be adopted depending on the width of the chimney. If the chimney is very wide, you may have to climb using a handhold and foothold on either side by straddling the chimney. Any effective chimneying technique usually entails a considerable amount of shuffling and all manner of handholds and footholds, but mostly those that require pressure to remain effective.

OFF-WIDTH

An off-width crack is like a chimney but you can't get your body completely inside it. The ascent of such features will nearly always involve a struggle and won't be every climber's forte!

To climb an off-width crack effectively you'll need to use imagination to jam arms and legs in the crack. It's always worth scrabbling around inside the crack to see if there are any handholds or footholds that might aid progress. Always wear plenty of clothing when climbing off-widths, particularly when the rock is extremely rough.

← **Chimneys are 'classically' climbed using back and foot technique. The climber leans back on one side of the chimney and moves the feet up as high as is comfortable. The hands are placed behind, flat on the wall and the body pushed upwards while maintaining forceful pressure on the opposite wall with the feet. Once the move has been completed a resting position in the chimney can be had prior to repeating the process. It's preferable to wear slightly more protective clothing than the climber illustrated in this photo.**

↓ **If a chimney is too wide to back and foot, it may be straddled across its width. Whatever technique of chimneying is required, always try to find handholds that might be used to gain advantage.**

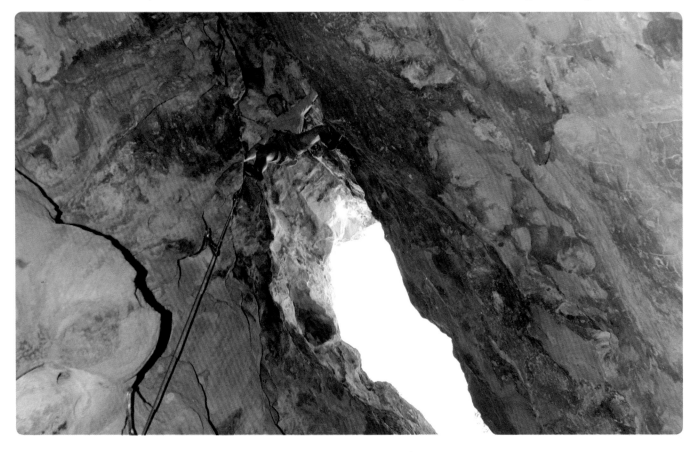

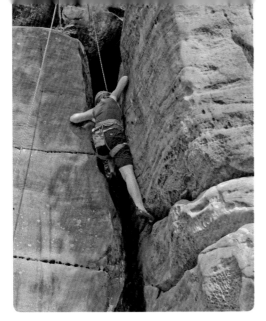

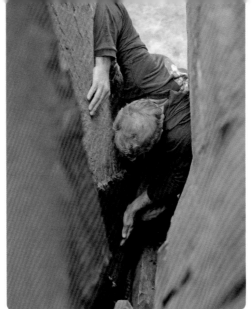

← **This is a
much more fierce off-width that
offers very little comfort.**

⬇ **Moving sideways across
the rock is called traversing,
which may utilise all manner of
handholds and footholds.**

⬆ **An off-width is a chimney that's too wide to jam but too narrow to get
comfortably into. Here it would be possible to get into the chimney but
it would be extremely tight. Sensibly the climber has decided to attempt
a combination of techniques, but most notably her hands are used on
sideways pulling handholds and are worked in opposition to each other to
provide the security needed to ascend. This also allows her to remain on the
outside of the chimney.**

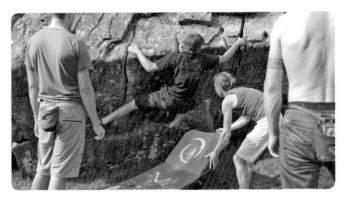

TRAVERSING

Moving sideways or diagonally across a rock face is called traversing.
Many boulder problem sequences are traverses that link a number
of sequential moves together to create a boulder problem. There
are also climbs that traverse cliffs and these are normally called girdle
traverses. When you traverse a rock face you use all of the various
types of handholds and footholds.

BRIDGING

Among the many features of rock faces are the types called grooves
and corners. One of the accompanying photos shows an excellent
example of a corner; a groove is simply a shallow version of a corner.

Very occasionally corners and grooves may be climbed just using a
crack feature deep in the corner itself but usually it's more comfortable
to climb by straddling the corner with the feet. In this manner the
climber is often able to fashion a resting position after every move and
may even be able to take both hands off the rock to arrange running
belays on the lead or to take them out when following a pitch.

The full gamut of footholds can be used, from smears to edges, and
the same wide range applies to handholds; pressure handholds are
particularly useful. Some of the more difficult corner and groove climbs
may not present any positive handholds or footholds and the rock
feature may only be climbed using smears and pressure holds.

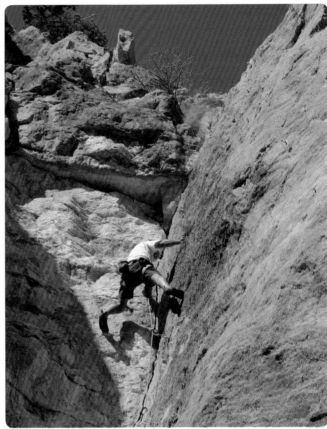

→ **Corners such as this feature are best climbed by a combination of
laybacking moves interspersed with bridging across the corner, when you
might even be able to arrange a hands-off rest. Some corner or groove
features can only be climbed by bridging; handholds and footholds may be
varied and plentiful, or sparsely placed and almost imaginary. The most
difficult climbs that ascend corners or grooves may involve only a series of
palming or pressure handholds and smears for the feet.**

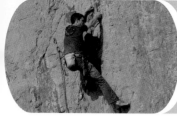

ADVANCED TECHNIQUES

The following techniques are generally too advanced for the beginner but are included for completeness.

DYNO

A dyno is the term used for a technique where the climber leaps for a handhold. It's a very powerful move that needs to be executed with precision and total confidence.

An example of a dyno is where the climber might be hanging on to two massive handholds just below the top of a climb. The feet are brought up as high as possible towards the hands and with a combination of an almighty push with both feet and simultaneously letting go with one or both hands the climber projects himself

upwards. You need to be sure that the handhold you're aiming for is a good one and that you have determined its exact location.

Extreme variations exist on difficult boulder problems and climbs where the dyno move is made for a handhold that might be judged only just viable.

⬇ **A dyno is a very dynamic move best attempted for the first time close to the ground on an indoor bouldering wall. It's extremely powerful and requires full commitment and confidence. There are climbs where climbers might make a jump for a handhold but it's usually done as a lunge in desperation to reach a good handhold – a dyno is much more calculated and deliberate.**

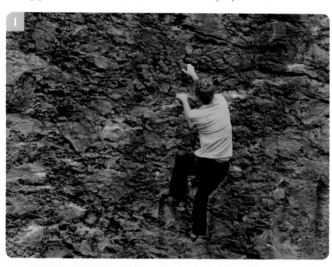

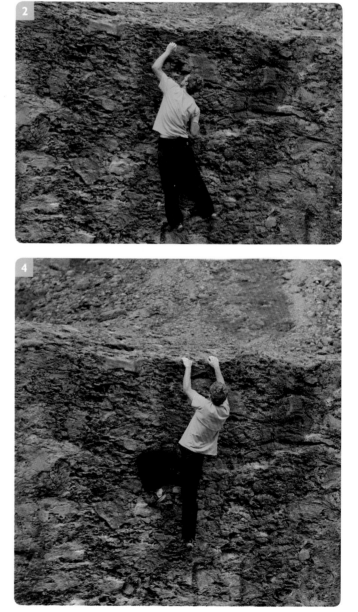

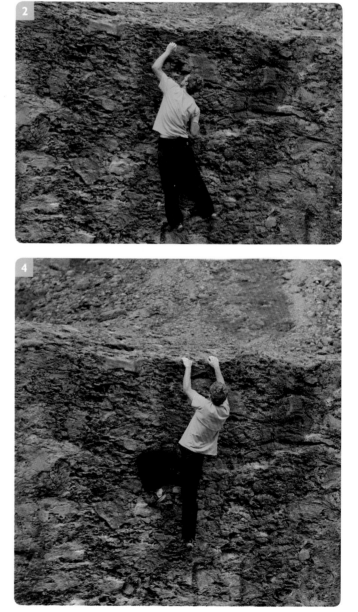

→ Heel hooking is a fairly advanced technique, but if you boulder to learn skills it's very useful to understand how effective a heel hook can be as a 'third handhold'. The climber on this overhanging rock face is able to relieve some of the weight on his arms by hooking his left heel on the horizontal break.

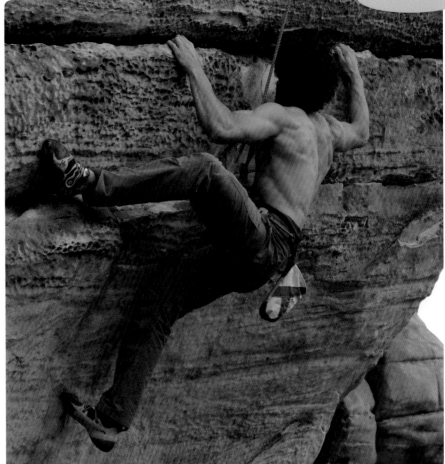

HEEL HOOKS

Heel hooks are used most often as a sort of 'third handhold' to help take some body weight off the arms and maintain a particular position, enabling the climber to reach for a higher handhold. A heel hook, which requires a certain amount of agility to use effectively, is commonly used to overcome a roof or overhang where the climber will hang limpet-like below the overhang, throw up a foot and hook the heel over a ledge or edge on or above the lip of the overhang. By sharing body weight between the heel hook and one handhold, the other hand can reach for a higher handhold, enabling the climber to pull the whole body around the overhang. It's a strenuous technique best mastered on a boulder problem at the climbing wall before trying it on a climb.

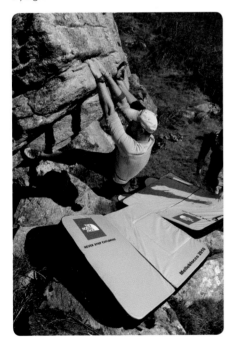

⬆ Surmounting an overhang: flat handholds and a heel hook to take some of the strain.

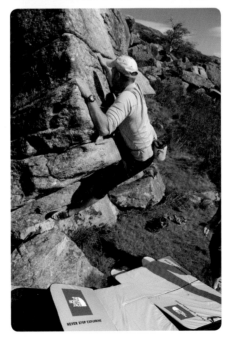

⬆ Reaching for higher handholds: this will allow you to pull body weight over the heel hook, transforming it into a foothold, albeit one that's tucked right under you. The climber then rocks over so that much of his weight is taken on the right foot.

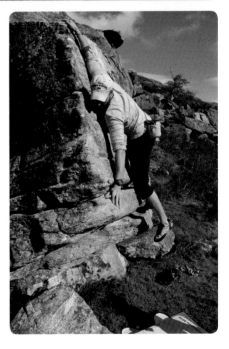

⬆ Push up hard on the right foot and move the right hand up over the top for a flat, rounded edge. The left hand is converted to a palming pressure hold to help push the body weight over the lip of the overhang.

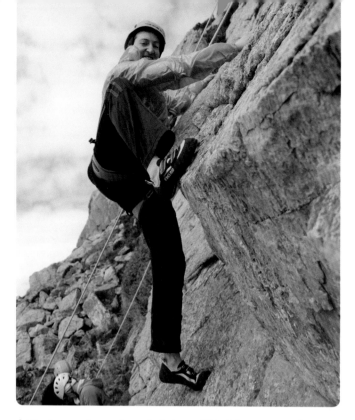

← Occasionally in climbing you may need to make a high step up. How high will largely depend on your flexibility but more importantly on the availability of handholds to help pull yourself up.

ROCKOVER

A rockover is any move where the climber makes a moderate-to-high step on to a foothold and needs to utilise mainly the powerful leg muscles in order to stand up on it. Handholds, if they exist, are usually some kind of sideways pulling hold and will be greatly appreciated.

KNEE BAR

A knee bar is where the lower part of the leg, including the knee, is used to help hold position on a climb or boulder problem. The accompanying photo taken at an indoor climbing wall is an extreme version of a double knee bar used on an almost horizontal roof. Such a position will relieve an enormous amount of strain from the arms. In the other photo, a single knee is wedged in a large limestone pocket, with the foot on the lower edge and the knee jammed inside the upper lip. A good knee bar will enable the climber to rest weary arms for a short while.

⬇ On steep rock experienced climbers will look for ways to relieve strain on their arms. With the knee-bar position illustrated here the climber has both feet on a large foothold and is using the feature to wedge his knees beneath. This is a radical position to find yourself in but serves to illustrate the infinite possibilities of using features on a wall or crag to your advantage.

⬇ A more straightforward knee bar is where the climber has one foot in the bottom of the hole and is able to insert the lower part of the leg and wedge the knee against the top of the hole. This will be a very effective resting position.

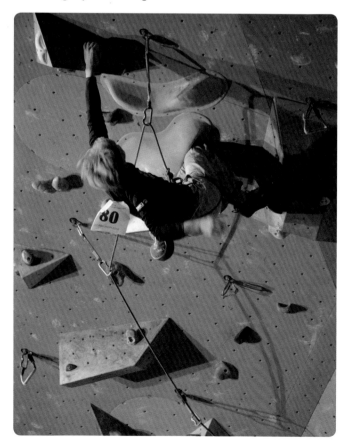

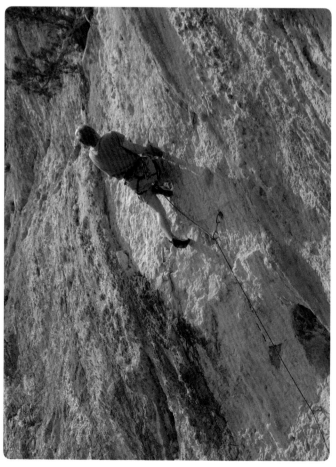

COUNTER-BALANCE OR 'FLAGGING'

Rock climbing is a dynamic and sometimes gymnastic sport, particularly beyond beginner level. Some of the techniques used on difficult climbs can be employed equally effectively at all levels of difficulty. The counter-balance move is particularly useful.

If, on an open expanse of rock, you find yourself faced with a move that relies on sideways holds for one or both hands (layaway or layback) there will be a tendency for the body to swing outwards like an opening door, a phenomenon named by climbers as 'barndooring'. When it happens it's quite alarming. To prevent barndooring, one leg can be stretched out sideways to counteract the effect. It doesn't always need to be placed on a foothold; simply pushing it to one side and resting it against the rock may be sufficient.

➔ **In order to counteract a barndooring effect, this climber has flagged his left leg across behind the other and out to the right. It's possible to imagine that without doing this his whole body would swing outwards to the right. Coincidentally the left foot is also on a foothold and the next move will be to take his weight on the left foot.**

⬇ **A leg placed out to the side allows the climber to maintain body weight directly over the other leg.**

⬊ **In this photo the climber has crossed hands in preparation for moving her left hand up for the jug handhold in the side of the flake above. It's important to develop your skill in 'reading the rock' in order to plan sequencing moves like this as it will save energy in the long term.**

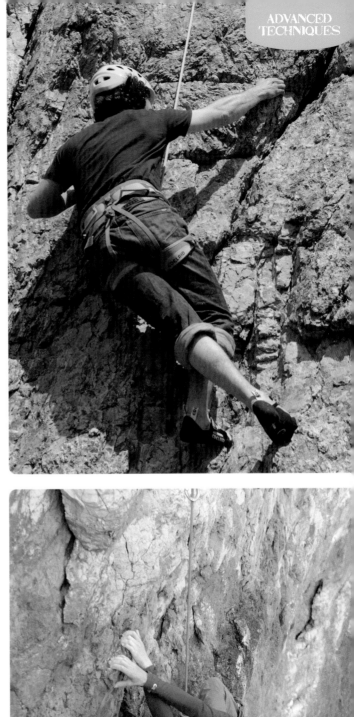

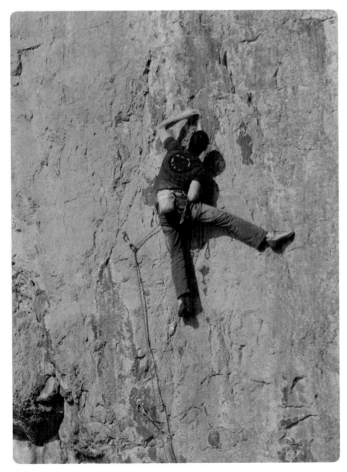

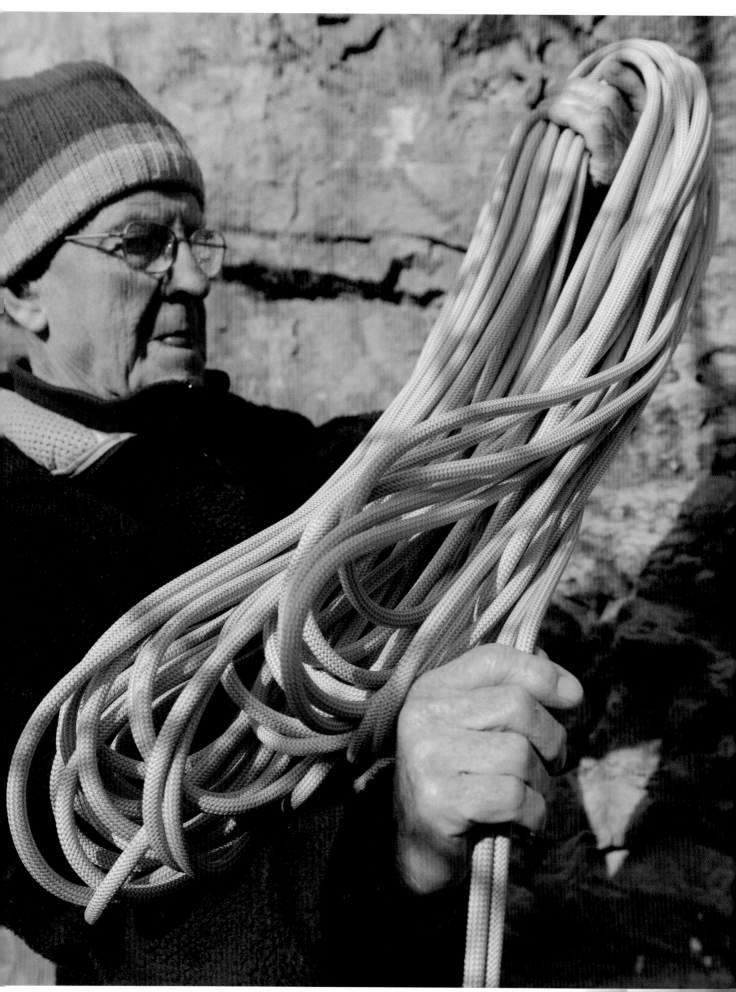

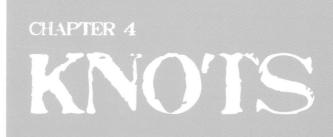

CHAPTER 4
KNOTS

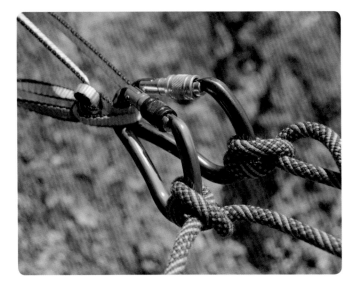

Always make sure that any knot you tie is recognisable – if you are unsure it's almost certainly incorrectly tied and must be redone.

For clarity, in this chapter we will divide knots into three categories: knots used for tying in to a rope; knots used for securing yourself to an anchor; and all other knots. Though there are very many knots illustrated in this chapter, climbers mainly use only two knots – one to tie in to the rope and another to secure to anchors.

Knot tying can be practised with a short piece of rope or cord. Whenever you tie a knot in a climbing situation, make sure that it's recognisable as the knot you intended to tie. If it isn't, the chances are that you have tied it incorrectly and it could be dangerous.

I'm a bit of a 'knot fascist' when it comes to tying knots and like to see them tied neatly as well as correctly!

The methods illustrated here for tying any knot are a suggestion only. Once you have mastered a particular knot it's likely that you'll develop your own technique for tying it. As long as the finished knot is correctly tied it doesn't really matter what sequence or method you use to get there.

⬇ **Sport climbers may get away with knowing very few knots or variations of knots but for Trad climbing you'll need to know a wide range for different applications.**

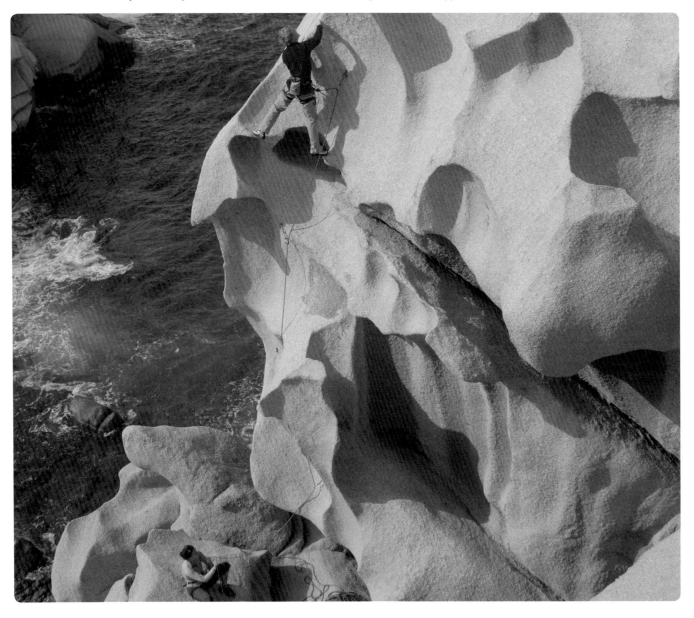

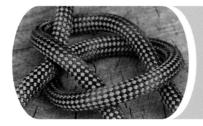

There are only two knots used to tie in to the rope – figure of eight and bowline – but there are also variations.

All climbing harnesses have specific tying-in points and each manufacturer provides clear instructions on how the rope should be secured to the harness. Though almost 99 per cent of harnesses use very similar systems to those illustrated here, the climber is always responsible for making sure that the rope is secured correctly according to manufacturer's recommendations.

There are two key points worth bearing in mind with all knots that are tied in the end of the rope:

◼ It's important to ensure that at least 4cm of rope end remains when you have completed the tie-in. The final securing knot is called a double-stopper knot and all end-of-rope tie methods must be secured this way.

◼ The final closed loop that joins the leg loops of your harness and the waist belt only needs to be large enough to push your fist through, or about the same size as the fixed belay loop that connects the two.

⬇⬈ **Rope tied through the correct part of the harness and linking the leg loops and belt together. One photo shows a compact tie-in loop and the second a more spacious one. Ideally the loop needs to be about the same size as the belay loop that's integral to the harness. The loop formed by the rope when it's tied in will be called the central loop throughout this book.**

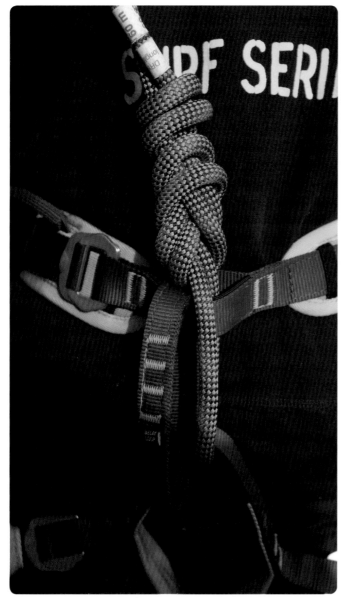

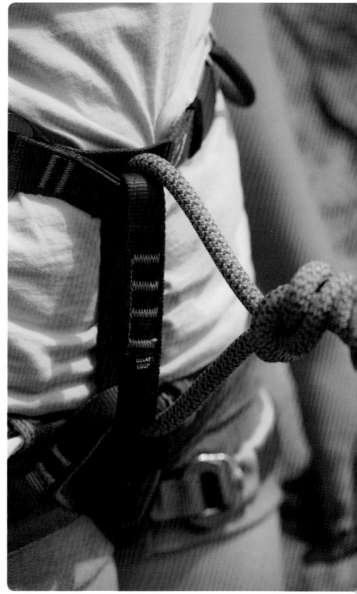

RETHREADED FIGURE OF EIGHT

This is without doubt the knot that's used most widely by climbers all around the world for tying in to the end of the rope. It's simple to tie, easy to recognise and very secure.

The positioning of the initial single figure of eight is critical, to ensure that there's sufficient rope to complete the finishing-off knot. This positioning will differ slightly according to the rope diameter: for 10mm rope the position is 90–100cm from the rope end, and for 8.5mm rope it's 85–95cm from the rope end.

When you have completed tying the knot make sure that all the strands of rope through the knot lie parallel to each other. The loop that's formed by the rope when you thread it through the leg loops and the waist belt of the harness should be about the same size as the fixed belay loop that links the two together.

The finishing-off knot is commonly known as the double-stopper knot. The extra rope remaining is used to tie this and it should be finished off so that it butts right up against the figure of eight knot.

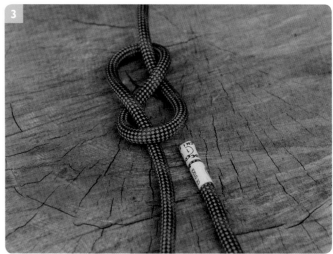

⬆ **Tie a single figure of eight knot 90–100cm from the end of the rope.**

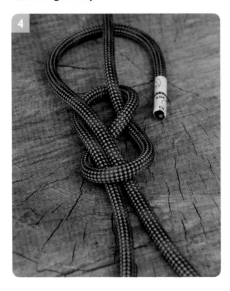

⬆ **If it makes it easier you can tie it close to the end and then move the knot along the rope.**

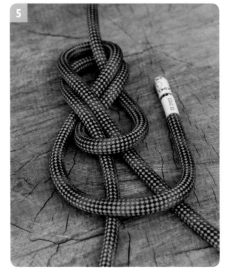

⬆ **Thread the rope up through the leg loops then the waist belt, ensuring that it goes through the correct parts of the harness as recommended by the manufacturer.**

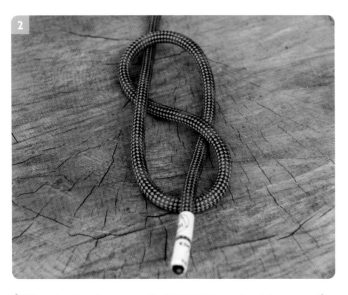

⬆ **Begin to re-trace the end back through the original figure of eight.**

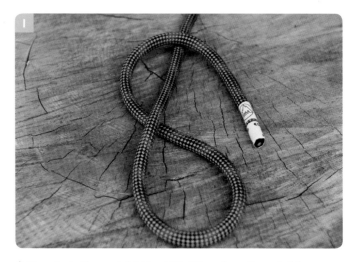

⬆ **Make sure you follow it neatly.**

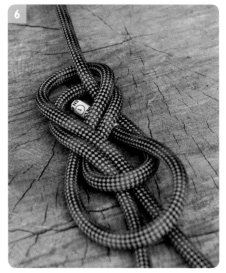

⬆ **Finally the end comes out of the knot and points away from you.**

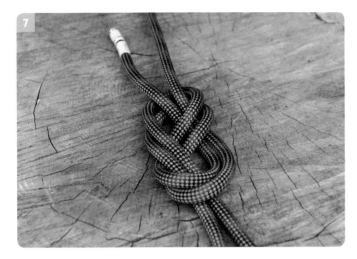

⬆ This photo shows only a short tail end. If you have positioned the figure of eight as suggested this tail end will be longer than that shown.

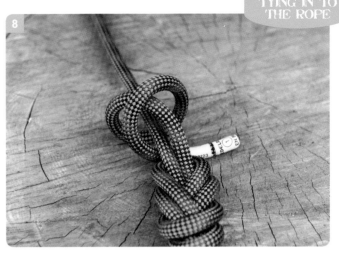

⬆ To complete the safety stopper knot spiral the end of rope around once...

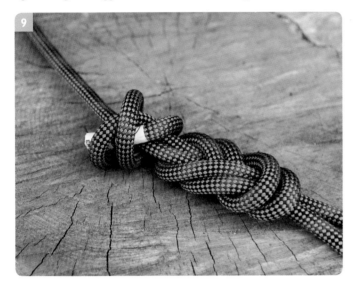

⬆ ...and a second time, then poke the rope end through the double loop.

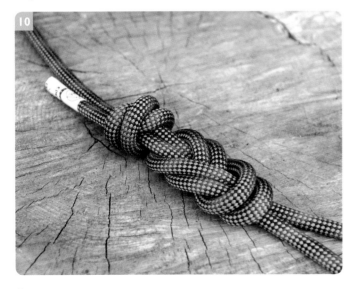

⬆ Pull everything tight and snug, making sure that the safety stopper knot sits right up against the figure of eight.

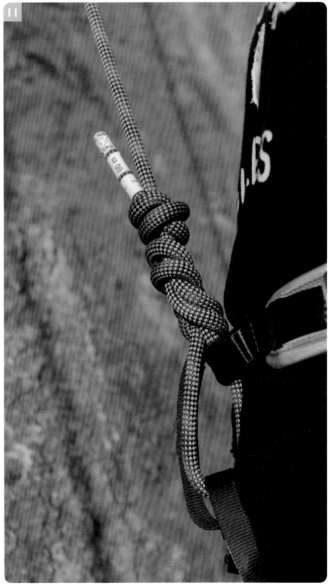

⬆ The completed knot.

BOWLINE

This is a more traditional knot for tying in to a rope. The bowline has one key advantage over the rethreaded figure of eight in that it's easier to untie after it has been subjected to a load, such as the force generated by a falling leader. It's very important to finish off a bowline with the final securing double-stopper knot, otherwise there's a heightened possibility that the knot may unravel during use. You must ensure that the double-stopper securing knot sits snugly up against the bowline itself.

The first sequence of photos shows the bowline tied with a single loop and the second sequence with a double loop. This second method is more secure than the first.

Bowline with single loop

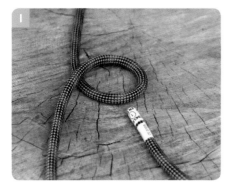

⬆ To begin with thread the end of the climbing rope up through the leg loops and the waist belt, making sure you do it exactly as the manufacturer recommends. Form a loop on the main climbing rope where it comes out from under the leg loops.

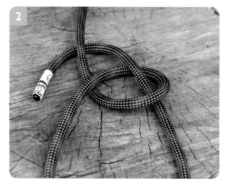

⬆ Take the end from above the waist belt and pass it through the loop from underneath.

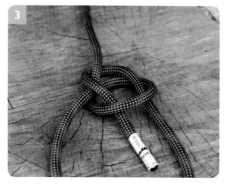

⬆ Take the end around the main rope and push it back through the loop.

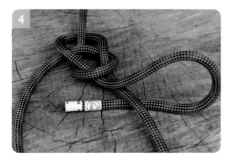

⬆ Now we need to tie a safety stopper knot, which is exactly the same knot used in the rethreaded figure of eight.

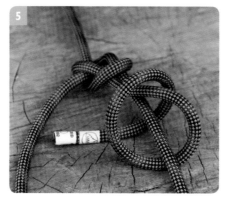

⬆ Make two turns around with the second turn on the bowline side.

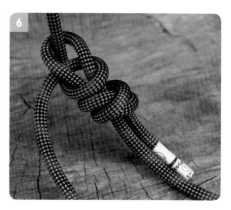

⬆ Pass the end through the two loops and pull it tight so that it fits snugly up against the main bowline knot.

Bowline with double loop

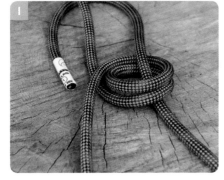

⬆ A safer version of the bowline is one where a double loop is formed right at the beginning of the process.

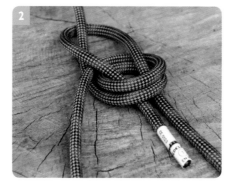

⬆ Bring the rope end up through the two loops, around the main rope and back down through the two loops.

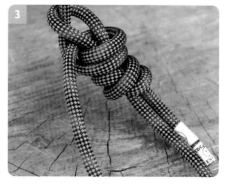

⬆ Finish off with a safety stopper knot.

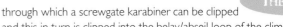
FIGURE OF EIGHT ON THE BIGHT

There will be occasions when it's desirable to secure yourself to the end of rope using a screwgate karabiner. This method is most often used, indoors or outdoors, when learning or when top-roping a single-pitch climb. It's also more convenient when several climbers need to ascend the same climb one after the other.

When completed, the figure of eight on a bight forms a small loop through which a screwgate karabiner can be clipped and this in turn is clipped into the belay/abseil loop of the climbing harness. Finally the locking sleeve of the karabiner must be screwed securely to prevent the rope detaching itself.

Begin by doubling the rope end so that you have a double length of around 75cm. The completed knot should have a closed loop no larger than the thickness of two fingers.

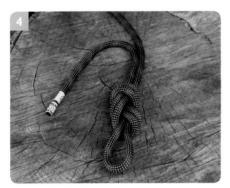

⬆ **The figure of eight on a bight is tied in the doubled rope end. The double length or bight needs to be around 75cm long. Begin by forming a loop as shown.**

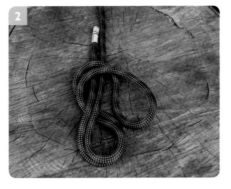

⬆ **Bring the closed end of the bight over the top…**

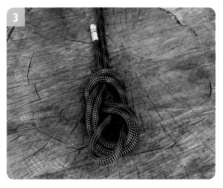

⬆ **…and pass it back through the first loop.**

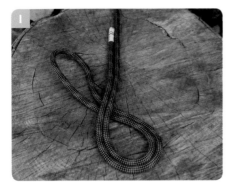

⬆ **You should have a small closed loop and around 30cm of tail end remaining.**

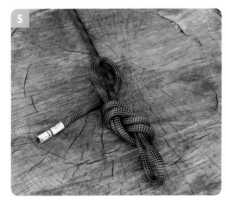

⬆ **Finish with a safety double stopper knot, as with the previous two knots.**

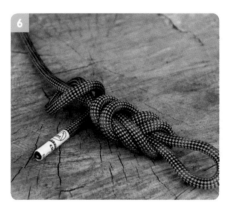

⬆ **Always make the second turn on the knot side.**

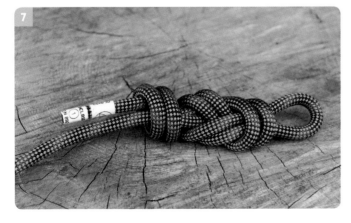

⬆ **Make sure that the stopper knot sits snugly up against the main figure of eight knot and that there's a good 5cm or so of tail end.**

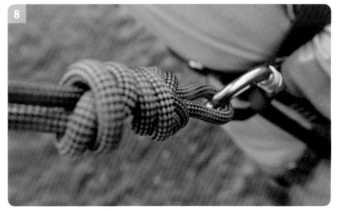

⬆ **The finished knot clipped directly to the harness belay loop with a screwgate karabiner securely fastened.**

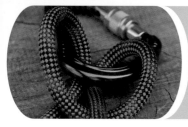

These are by far the most commonly used knots. Here the knots are simply illustrated and briefly explained; where they fit into the grand scheme of things is examined in the next chapter, which covers all aspects of safety.

CLOVE HITCH

This is a locking knot that can be easily adjusted to any length. When anchoring to the rock face it's secured around a karabiner, normally a screwgate variety. It can be quite difficult to undo after it has been subjected to a severe or continuous load.

The clove hitch can be tied in both rope and tape and there are several applications for the knot in a wide variety of climbing scenarios.

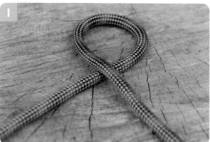

⬆ **Form a loop as shown.**

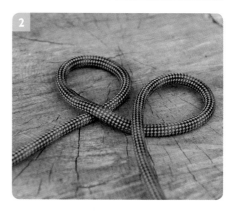

⬆ **Form a second loop in exactly the same way.**

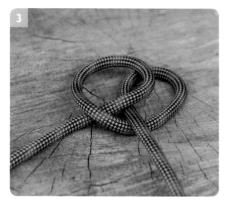

⬆ **Pass the right hand loop under the left.**

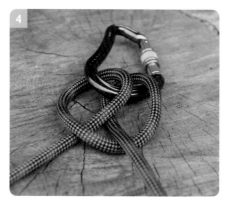

⬆ **Clip the two loops into a screwgate karabiner.**

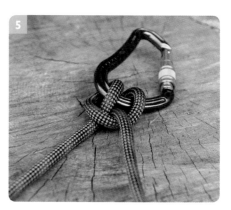

⬆ **Clinch the clove hitch tightly and screw up the sleeve of the screwgate karabiner so that it's locked.**

⬇ **There may be times when you'll appreciate the ability to tie a clove hitch with one hand, so here's a suggestion. It's much easier to tie with one hand when there's some tension in the rope.**

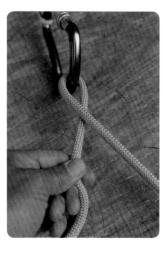
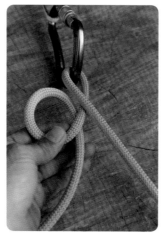
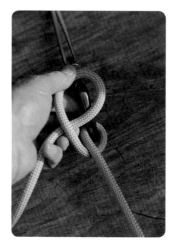
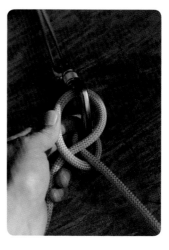

Rethreaded figure of eight

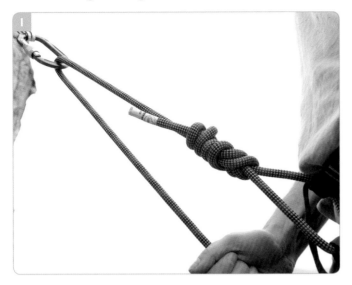

⬆ **The rethreaded figure of eight is a useful knot to have in your armoury of methods of securing to anchor points.**

FIGURE OF EIGHT ON THE BIGHT

The figure of eight on the bight can also be used for tying back into anchors as illustrated, though it's less easily adjusted than the clove hitch and should really only be used if the anchor point is within arm's reach.

RETHREADED DOUBLE FIGURE OF EIGHT

This is a very handy method of tying off the rope from an anchor point back into the harness if you find that you don't have a screwgate karabiner spare to tie back using a clove hitch.

This knot does require a fair bit of rope to tie safely as you must ensure that there's at least 35–40cm of spare tail sticking out of the tied knot to be sure that it's safe.

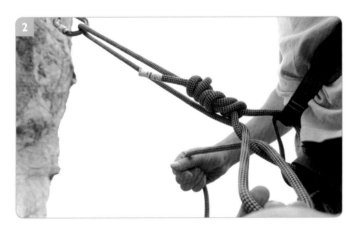

⬆ **Thread a loop of rope through the harness tie-in rope loop (central loop).**

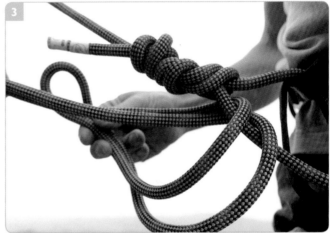

⬆ **Use the bight of rope to tie a figure of eight knot around itself.**

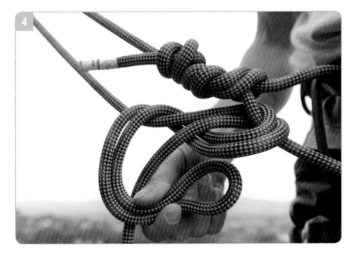

⬆ **Make sure that the knot you tie looks like the number 8.**

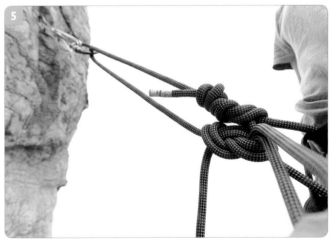

⬆ **The finished, secured knot needs to have a loop of rope of at least 45cm for safety.**

KNOTS 67

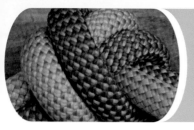

Though the previous two sections cover the knots that are most commonly used in climbing, there's a wide range of other knots to learn for particular climbing scenarios.

ITALIAN HITCH

This is a sliding friction knot and is most often used to lower a climber from above or for belaying a climber in ascent, again from above. It's included here because it's a quick method of safeguarding a climber on an easy section of climbing or scrambling that might be part of a multi-pitch climb.

The most frequent application for an Italian hitch is in what's termed a 'direct belay'. This differs from the more traditional way of belaying, using a belay device on the harness, in that it's used directly attached to an anchor. The simplest situation is a sling draped over a large flake or bollard of rock. A large pear-shaped (HMS) karabiner must be used for an Italian hitch because it allows the knot to flow freely in either direction. As the rope is attached directly to the anchor point any loading will be taken fully on the anchor, which, of course, must be 100 per cent sound.

The Italian hitch belay is very quick to implement in simple climbing scenarios and it's also surprisingly easy to hold a climber's weight when using an Italian hitch belay. The person operating the Italian hitch belay should be clipped into an anchor, stand directly below the Italian hitch belay and ideally wear gloves.

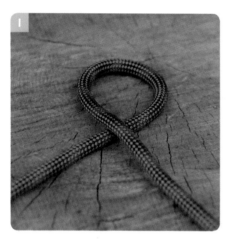

⬆ **The Italian hitch begins in exactly the same way as the clove hitch.**

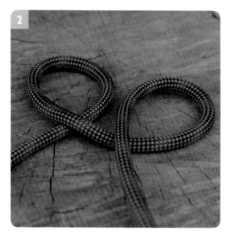

⬆ **This step is again the same as the clove hitch.**

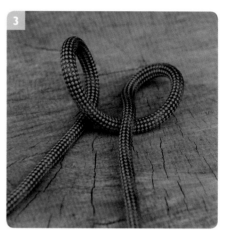

⬆ **Simply fold the two loops together – like closing a book.**

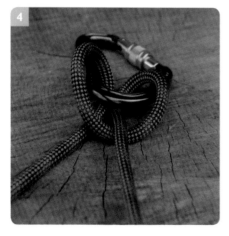

⬆ **Clip the two loops into a screwgate karabiner (HMS).**

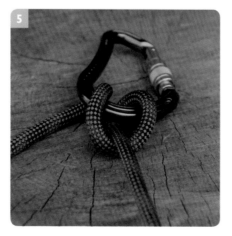

⬆ **Screw the locking sleeve tightly closed.**

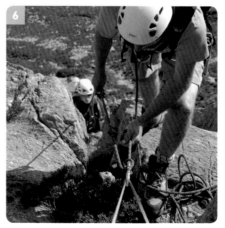

⬆ **A climber operates the Italian hitch to safeguard a companion. The Italian hitch is an emergency knot that can be used for a number of the situations discussed in more detail in Chapter 9.**

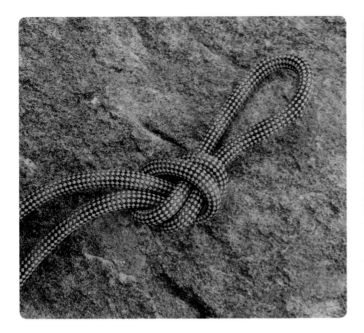

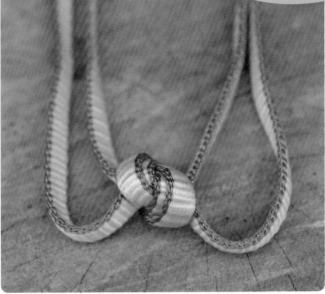

OVERHAND

There are two main uses for the overhand knot:

- When you use a sling to create a single attachment point to two or more anchors you will tie an overhand knot, using one of the slightly different methods shown in the accompanying photos.
- The overhand knot can be used effectively for tying together two ropes for a long double-rope abseil descent (see Chapter 8), but it's absolutely essential for safety that the two ropes are of the same diameter.

The overhand knot isn't commonly used for attaching yourself to a rope or an anchor. If you want to tie in to the rope and attach it to your harness the figure of eight is better and just as easy to tie. The overhand knot is perfectly strong enough but is very difficult to untie after it has been subjected to a load.

The overhand knot is also the basis for the tape knot or ring bend (see overleaf).

The overhand knot is one of the simplest there is, here shown tied in three situations: a bight of the rope (above left); the mid-point of a tape sling (above) and a doubled tape (below).

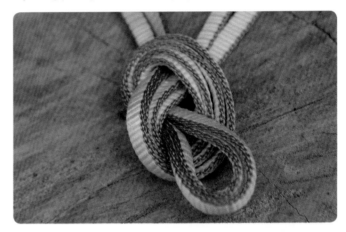

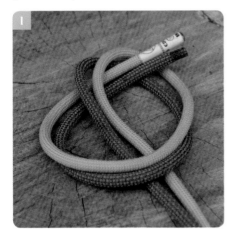

⬆ **An overhand knot tied in the ends of rope.**

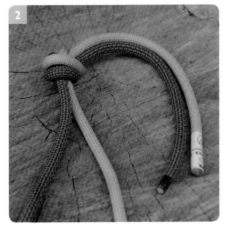

⬆ **Make sure that the knot is tied with at least 45cm of tail end of rope if you'll use it to join two ropes together.**

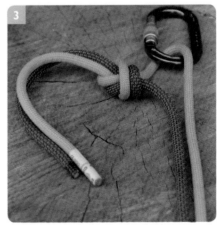

⬆ **Here the ropes are illustrated clipped through a karabiner such as might be used on a retrievable abseil (see Chapter 8).**

DOUBLE FISHERMAN'S

If you're a fisherman you'll already know how to tie this knot! It has two main applications in rock climbing:

■ To join two ends of rope together for abseiling.
■ To tie the ends of a rope when it's used for threading nuts or making rope slings.

The knot is basically a pair of double-stopper knots, one at each rope end tied around the other so that they slide together to butt securely against each other, so that they can't unravel.

It's vital to tie the knot correctly as illustrated. If you have tied it properly one side of the knot should feature four parallel and neatly fitting strands of rope and the other sides of the knot should snuggle up neatly against each other. It's important to leave at least 4cm of tail end sticking out of the knot, to allow for some slippage when the knot tightens up under load.

When joining two ropes together, the double fisherman's knot can be used with ropes of unequal diameter – unlike the overhand knot – as long as the difference in diameter is no more than a few millimetres.

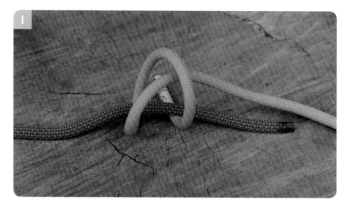

↑ **The double fisherman's knot is used to join together two ends of rope. It's basically two double safety stopper knots back to back.**

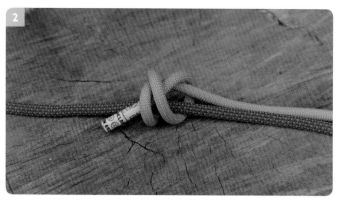

↑ **The first double safety stopper is tied in one direction around the second rope.**

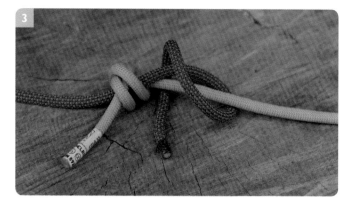

↑ **The second stopper is spiralled around the rope in the opposite direction from the first.**

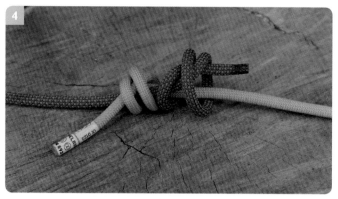

↑ **The ends of rope should come out of the knot on opposite sides of it.**

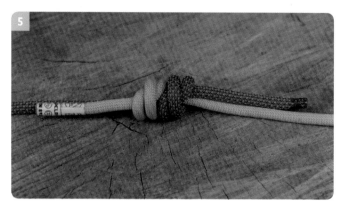

↑ **The stoppers should fit snugly into each other as illustrated.**

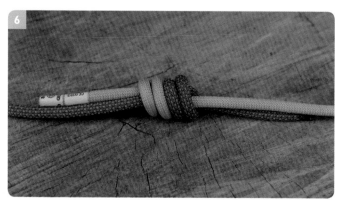

↑ **The other side should present four parallel strands of rope.**

REEF KNOT

This knot only has one use in rock climbing. For abseiling, it's often inserted into the rope between a double fisherman's knot where it prevents the double fisherman's becoming over-tight and difficult to release.

The simple reef knot is easy to tie but if tied incorrectly it becomes a granny knot, which is exceedingly dangerous.

RING BEND OR TAPE KNOT

This knot can be used in both tape and rope. It's very simple to tie but all the strands of rope must lie parallel and fit snugly into each other. When tying in tape, ensure that there are no twists in the tape and that the knot is tightened securely before use.

It's rare nowadays to use knotted tape slings (factory-stitched slings are much more common), but they can be useful in certain climbing situations. The most significant purpose is when you need to rig an anchor to retreat from a climb and wish to leave behind a sling from which you can abseil.

For safety, a Dyneema sling should be knotted using a double fisherman's knot rather than a tape knot, to avoid any possibility of slippage and consequent danger.

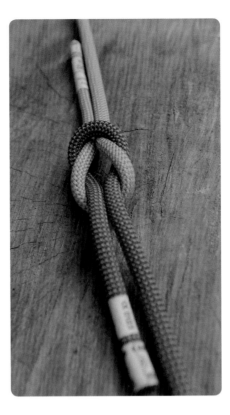

← **A reef knot – the only way to tie this incorrectly results in a granny knot and is extremely dangerous.**

⬇ **A double fisherman's knot tied with a reef knot in between is a very safe knot for joining two ropes together for an abseil. The knot is much easier to untie after several people have abseiled on the ropes.**

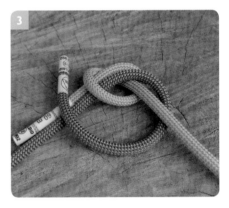

Ring bend or tape knot

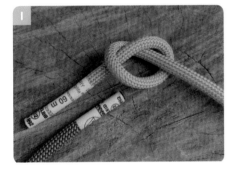

⬆ **The ring bend or tape knot can be tied in both tape and rope. Tie an overhand in the end of the rope or tape about 10–12cm in from the end.**

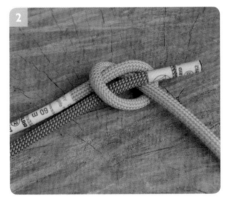

⬆ **Take the other rope end and thread it through the middle of the first knot.**

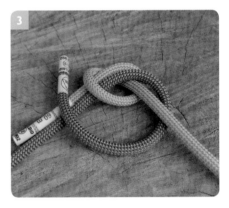

⬆ **Trace the line of the original knot.**

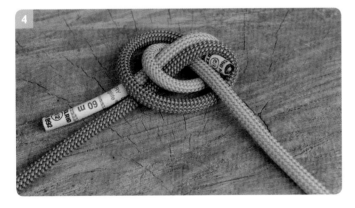

⬆ **Continue to trace that line.**

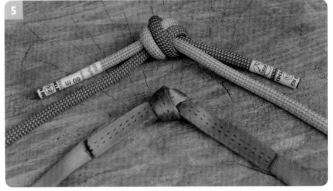

⬆ **This shows the finished knot in both tape and rope. Always ensure that the knot is tight and there's at least 10cm of spare tail on each end.**

PRUSIK KNOTS

'Prusiking' is the term applied to the manner in which a fixed rope can be climbed. The climber uses two slings of cord, one attached to the sit harness and the other for a foot loop. The Prusik knot is tied around the fixed rope and when tied correctly the knot will grip on to the rope. When the climber needs to slide the knot up the rope it's easily slackened and moved; the climber will alternately move the sit loop and the foot loop in order to ascend. Chapter 9 illustrates various emergency rope ascent methods.

A Prusik loop is formed from accessory cord, usually of 5mm diameter but 6mm is better. Each loop is made from a 1.5m length of cord and the ends are joined using a double fisherman's knot with at least 2.5cm of tail end after the knot is really tightened.

There are a number of different styles of Prusik knot but essentially three types will suffice:

■ **Original Prusik** This simply comprises two turns of the Prusik loop around the fixed rope and then threaded back through itself. This knot is used only to ascend the rope. The knot cannot be released while it's loaded and this makes it particularly secure when ascending a fixed rope. On completion of the knot it's vital to ensure that all the strands lie parallel to each other, otherwise the

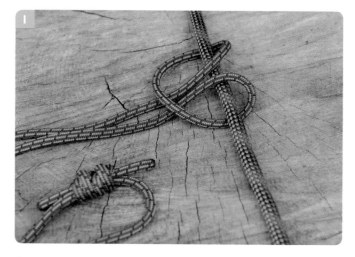

⇧ **Pass the loop around the back of the rope and thread it through itself. Keep the knotted part of the loop at one end.**

knot may not grip on to the rope. If you discover that two turns are insufficient for grip, a third turn can be introduced.

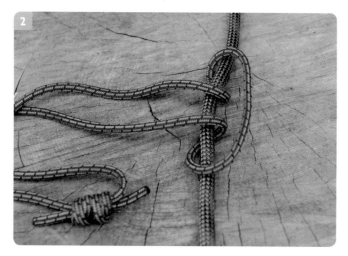

⇧ **Repeat the wrap-around a second time, again passing it back through on itself.**

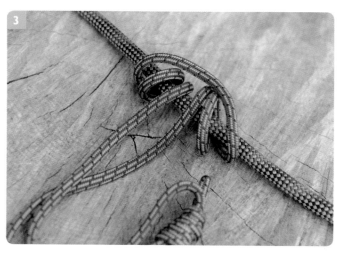

⇧ **Begin to pull the wraps around tight.**

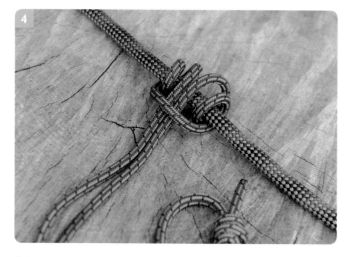

⇧ **As you tighten the wraps, make sure that the strands lie parallel to each other, without twist.**

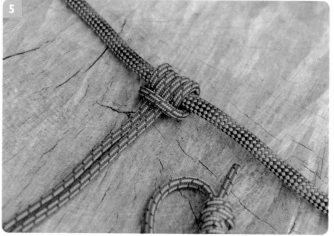

⇧ **The finished knot should present a clean, neat profile as illustrated.**

French Prusik

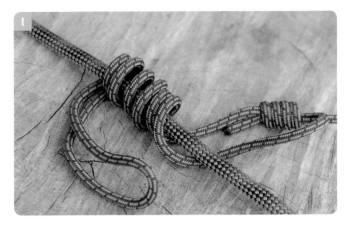

⬆ Take your Prusik loop and hold the knotted part in your hand. Spiral the rest of the loop up the rope about five times.

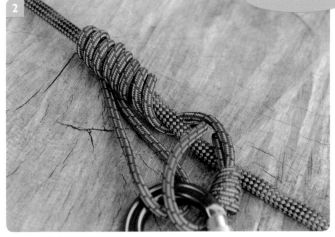

⬆ Bring the closed loop back to the knotted end and clip both loops into a screwgate karabiner.

■ **French Prusik** Also called a Marchand knot and sometimes described as an Autobloc, this type of Prusik knot can also be used to ascend a fixed rope, but it's more commonly used to protect the climber on an abseil. If the abseiler accidentally (or deliberately) lets go of the controlling rope, this knot will grip on to the rope (see Chapter 8). The French Prusik offers one big advantage over the original Prusik in that it can be released while under load, but this attribute also makes it an inappropriate knot to use for ascending a rope in certain situations, particularly in rescue.

■ **Klemheist** This other handy Prusik knot to learn has similar attributes to the French Prusik, but is a little more difficult to release when under load. Its biggest advantage is that it can be used very effectively in a tape sling wrapped around the rope – which might be handy if you forget, or accidentally drop, your Prusik loop.

Klemheist

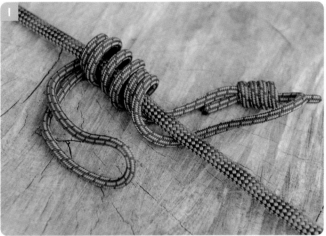

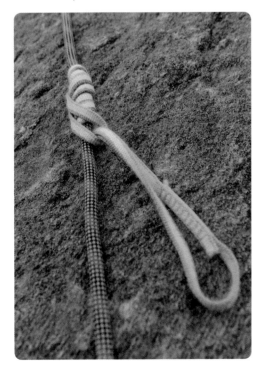

⬅ It's also possible to use the Klemheist knot in a tape sling. Narrow slings are particularly good for this. Try to make sure that all the strands of tape lie as neatly as possible.

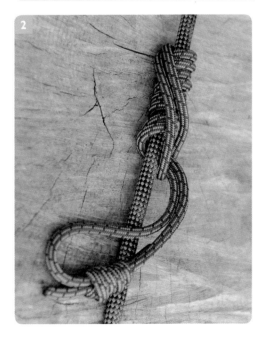

⬆ The Klemheist begins in a similar way to the French Prusik...

⬅ But instead of clipping two end loops together the lower loop is passed through the top loop as shown.

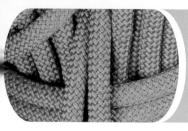

COILING A ROPE

Two methods of coiling a rope are explained here, though the first is very much the more practical and commonly used.

ALPINE-STYLE DOUBLE COILING

When coiled correctly the rope can be slung over the back and the spare tail ends of rope used to secure it so that it can be carried like a rucksack.

This method of coiling to carry the rope is particularly useful at the top of a multi-pitch climb where you have a long walk or scramble back to the foot of the crag to reunite yourself with any gear you may have left at the bottom of the climb.

TRADITIONAL LOOP COILING

Though rarely used nowadays, this method of coiling a rope is included for completeness and because it can be a very good way to carry a rope for particular situations.

When you coil traditionally your arms do tend to become a little pumped up, particularly with a very long rope, but another way to achieve the same result is to coil the rope around your neck. The whipping method used to finish off the rope securely, so that it doesn't unravel, should be wrapped snugly around all of the coils.

Coiling a rope

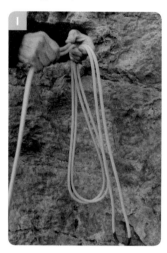

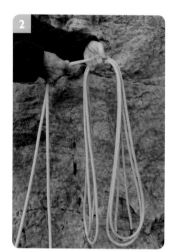

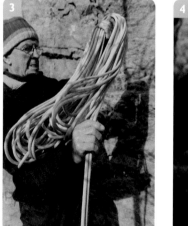

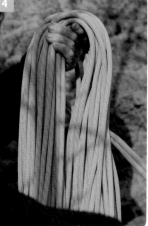

⬆ Find the mid-point of the rope, hold the doubled rope about 80cm from the 'end' and begin lapping the rope over your hand.

⬆ When you have about 2.5m of rope left to coil, grip all the lapped coils firmly and begin wrapping the remaining rope around all the laps (this is sometimes referred to as the 'whipping').

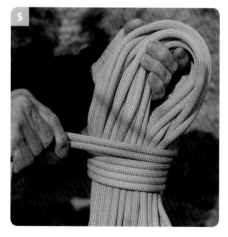

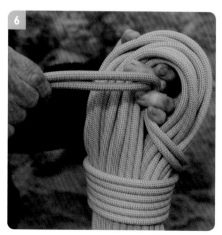

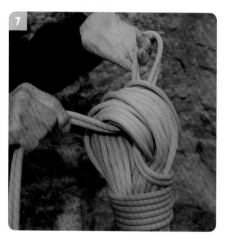

⬆ Do three or four turns...

⬆ ...and then push the rope into the holding hand.

⬆ Pull a loop all the way through – it needs to be a bit bigger than fist size.

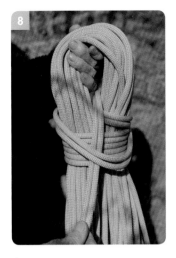

⬆ **Now for the tricky bit – without dropping all the coils, let the loop fall over the top…**

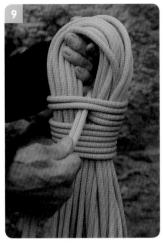

⬆ **Drop it to the level of the 'whipping' and tighten all the strands of 'whipping' snugly around the main body of coils.**

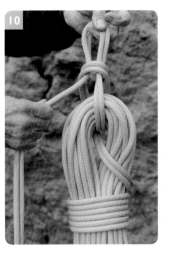

⬆ **An alternative method to secure the whipping is illustrated here. Instead of looping over the top of the coils, take the double strands and thread them through the loop.**

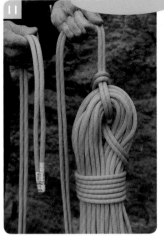

⬆ **Pull them all the way through to cinch tight.**

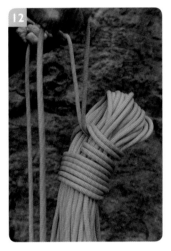

⬆ **The spare tails of rope enable you to carry the rope like a 'backpack'.**

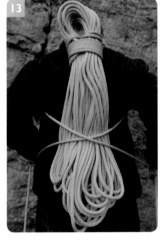

⬆ **Sling the rope over your back with one strand of tail end over each shoulder, and cross these two strands over the back of the coiled rope.**

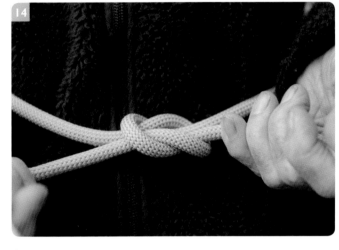

⬆ **Bring the ends around the front and secure using a reef knot.**

ROPE BAG

For a single climbing rope used at the climbing wall or for single-pitch sport climbing, a rope bag is the most sensible option. No coiling of the rope is required: the rope can simply be piled or lapped neatly into the bag, the bag rolled up, and carried as a rucksack or shoved inside your climbing pack.

Most rope bags feature loops for tying each end of the rope so that you can find them easily. An alternative method for easy location is to tie a chunky knot in each end of the rope.

A great thing about rope bags is that they include a large sheet or tarp that can be spread over the ground so the rope can be kept clean, and also provides you with a handy mat to stand on or sit on while you put on your climbing shoes.

When climbing on double or half ropes, it isn't usual to carry them in a rope bag though there's no reason why not.

A rope bucket is also an extremely useful piece of kit, particularly on a hanging belay stance above the sea.

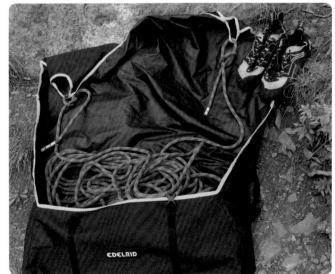

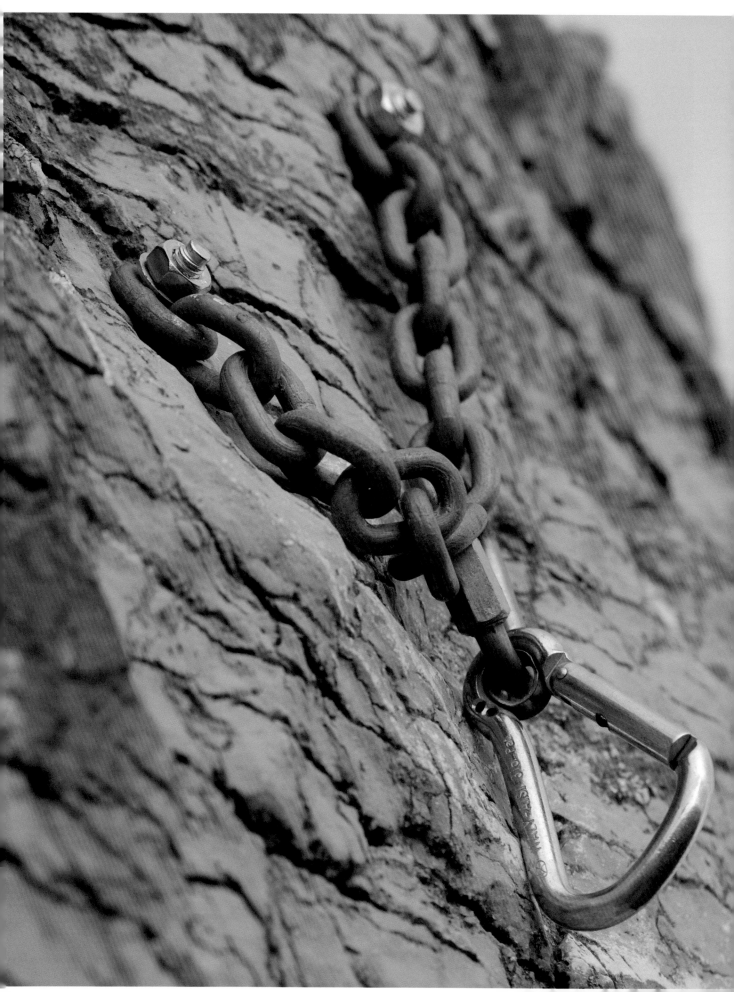

PROTECTION

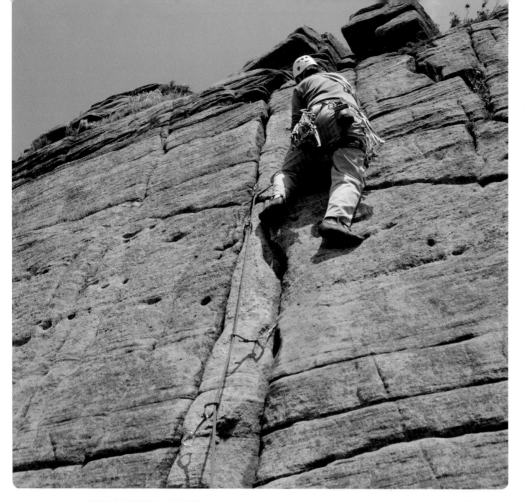

Protection is the collective term for all manner of gadgets and gizmos used to make climbers safe on the rock. In this chapter we'll look at various options, show how they each work individually, and how they might be used in conjunction with each other in the overall safety system.

← **Crack protection arranged by the leader on a trad climb. Each piece of protection needs to be carefully placed with the consideration that it might need to hold a fall.**

↓ **Crack-protection devices are often used to create anchors for securing the climbing party during the various stages or pitches of a climb.**

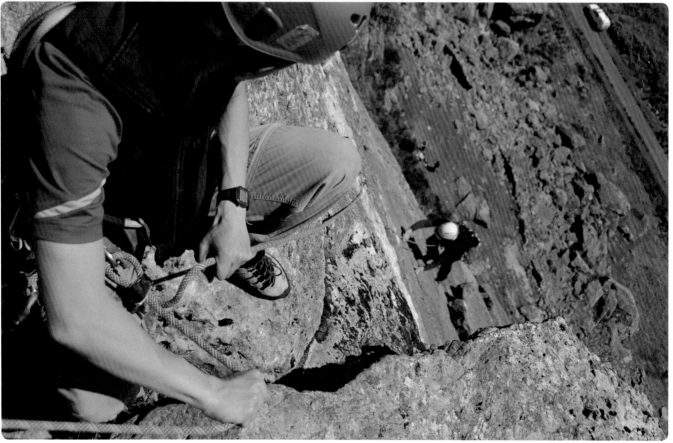

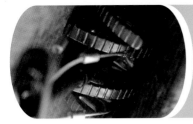

CRACK PROTECTION

Arranging safe and secure placements of crack protection is one of the trickiest aspects of learning about rock climbing. The basic principle is simple enough: take a lump of metal and wedge it in a crack so that when it's loaded it can only become tighter within the crack. However, once you have grasped the essentials of crack protection, the real learning process takes place as you build up experience. Confidence to place secure gear may not come until you have actually loaded several placements and discovered that they will indeed hold a load.

To begin with it's a very good idea to practise as much as possible in secure situations close to the ground where poor placement won't result in injury. A good procedure is to find somewhere to put various placements in the rock and attach a rope to them to test how effective they are at holding a load. The security of placement for all crack protection is dependent on rock quality and on how much of the piece of protection is in contact with the rock.

Experiment with the many variations in placement to discover how they perform. Some placements are fairly obvious, but many are less so; what may seem an unlikely placement may well prove surprisingly effective. The variations are almost infinite so be prepared for a long learning process.

Don't just practise putting gear into cracks – practise getting it out too! Just because a piece of gear is difficult to extract doesn't always mean that it's a good placement.

→ **You can practise placing crack protection just off the ground. Tying on to the rope as though you were leading a climb is useful when practising clipping into protection.**

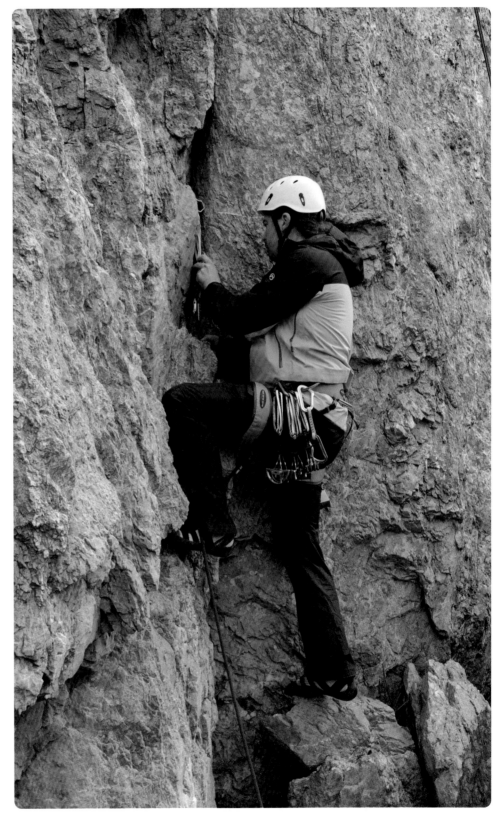

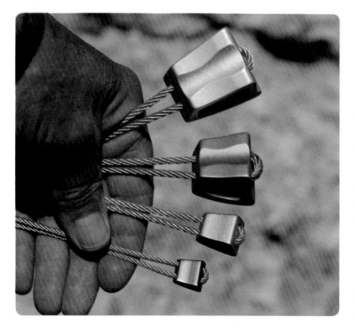

All crack protection is used either to protect the lead climber in an ascent or to create anchor points on ledges or stopping points, called 'belays' or 'stances'. Crack protection can also be used to create anchors at the top of an outcrop for bottom-rope or top-rope single-pitch climbing.

Most climbing protection equipment is categorised as 'passive', where devices – such as nuts or hexes – have no moving parts. 'Active' protection includes items that have moving parts, such as camming devices, also known as SLCDs (Spring-Loaded Camming Devices).

WEDGE-SHAPED NUTS

The simplest placement of all is to use a wedge-shaped nut in a crack that tapers downwards. The larger the wedge-shaped nut, the more contact it has with surrounding rock and the tighter it fits – the better it will be!

← **A variety of wedge-shaped nuts on wire slings. A range of sizes must be carried and sometimes climbers will carry two of each size on more difficult climbs.**

⬇ **A DMM Dragon camming device: sizes of cams vary from minute to very large and incredibly expensive.**

⬇ **A perfectly placed wedge-shaped nut: a tapering crack where each side of the nut is in contact with rock is about as good as it gets.**

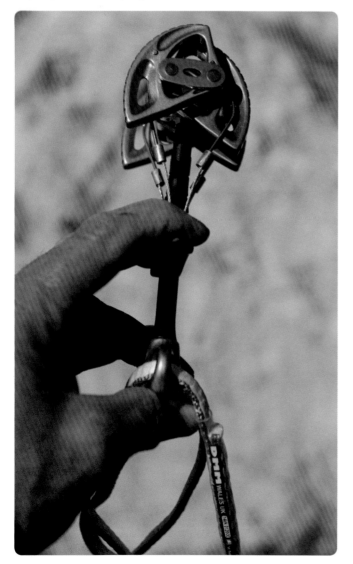

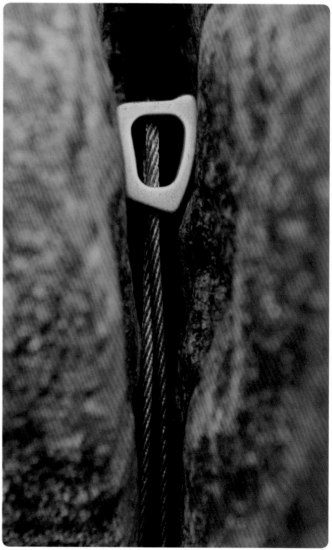

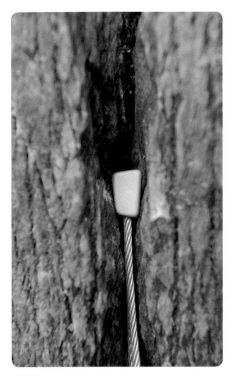

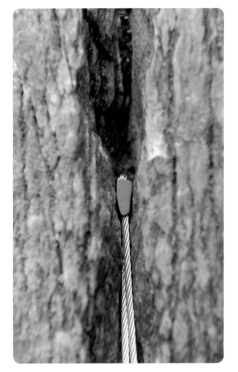

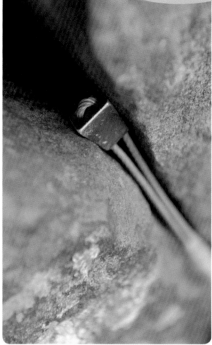

⬆ Though this nut will lock more tightly into the crack with a downwards force, it's a poor placement because not all of it is in contact with rock, and therefore could easily work loose and might fall out.

⬆ A more secure placement is achieved in the same crack with a smaller nut, which is less likely to come out accidentally – though there isn't so much leeway for tightening into the crack under a load.

⬆ Wedge-shaped and hex-shaped nuts can be placed in a crack along their widest profile; the same principles of nut to rock contact apply.

Different manufacturers offer slightly varying shapes and features along the same wedge-shaped principle. Choosing one brand over another is difficult as all do an excellent job.

Judging correctly first time what size nut will go in a particular crack can sometimes be difficult even for experienced climbers. A good tactic is to carry bunches of wired nuts of similar size on a single karabiner; this way, if your first choice of nut doesn't quite fit, you almost

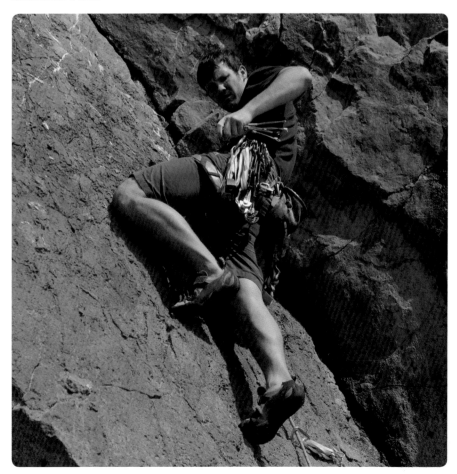

➜ You may not get the right-sized nut for a particular crack at the first attempt, but as you gain experience it'll become easier; even highly experienced climbers don't get it right first time. To help make the right choice as efficiently as possible, nuts of a similar size range are carried in a bunch on a single karabiner.

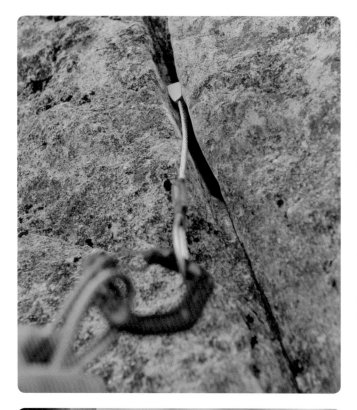

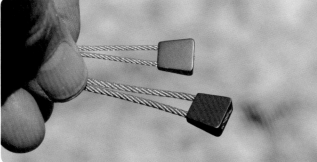

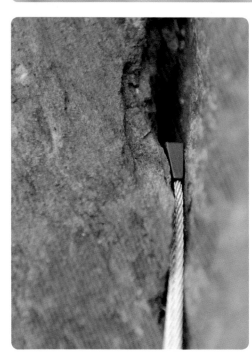

↑ **Micro-wires aren't essential for easier climbs where wider cracks for more substantial crack protection abound.**

← **This micro-wire is very well seated, with room for tightening further into the crack under a load.**

← **Whenever you place a nut in a crack, leave it attached to the bunch and give the whole thing a sharp downward tug in the direction of any potential load.**

instantly have access to one size bigger or smaller. We look at this in more detail in Chapter 7.

Whenever you place a nut, wedge-shaped or otherwise, it needs to be seated using a firm tug. A good method is to hold the whole bunch from which you have selected your chosen nut and pull sharply downwards in the same direction you think a load might come from.

All wedge-shaped nuts are numbered by size. There have been some attempts to standardise sizing across the range of manufacturers so that each number designation is very similar in size across the board. Size numbers range from 00 to 1 for micro wires and from 2 to 11 or 12 for the larger sizes.

Most nuts are slung with wire that features a manufactured swaged joint. Most wire is of 3mm diameter, which is exceptionally strong, but very tiny 'micro-wires' may only be 1mm thick or less.

↓ **For use as running belays to protect the leader, wire-slung nuts must always be attached to the rope via a quickdraw or extender; when used for creating anchors they can be clipped directly.**

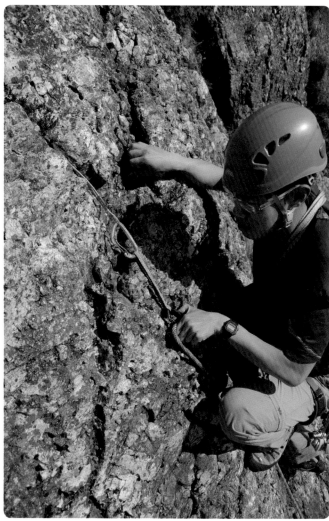

Micro-wires are particularly dependent for their security on rock quality and they rely on a tapered crack that suits the size almost perfectly for a sound placement. It's unlikely that even a perfectly placed micro-wire can sustain as severe a loading as a larger, similarly shaped nut.

When wired nuts are used as running belays (runners) to protect the leader, it's necessary to attach the rope via a quickdraw, which acts as a hinge to the placement. If the rope were to be clipped directly into the wire using a snaplink karabiner, the friction created as the rope runs through the krab would almost certainly lever the wire sling up and down. This could easily loosen the nut placement and alter its configuration, and sometimes it might even lift the nut out. If this happens to occur at a crucial safety point for the lead climber, it has potentially grave consequences.

It's possible to purchase unwired nuts and thread them on a rope or tape sling. This isn't commonly done nowadays, but this system has one advantage over wired nuts. As a rope or tape sling is considerably more flexible than the wired variety, it's possible to negate the need for a quickdraw extender when used as a running belay.

HEXES

Six-sided nuts like irregular hexagons have been used in rock climbing for decades. The concept of differing lengths and angles for the sides of a nut has its origins in the parallel-sided cracks commonly found in

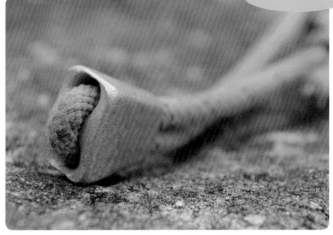

⬆ **A trusty old MOAC – one of the very first specifically-made nuts produced for climbing protection. This is an original.**

◤ ⬇ **Using a nut key to extract crack protection is good practice too. A troublesome and firmly stuck nut can often be loosened with a firm tap from below. Occasionally you may need to loosen a nut by wheedling it around from above. If you can get it to move it will come out…**

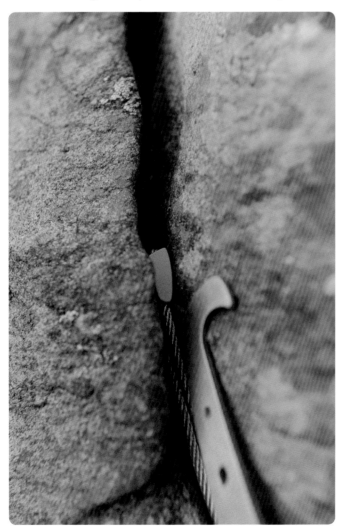

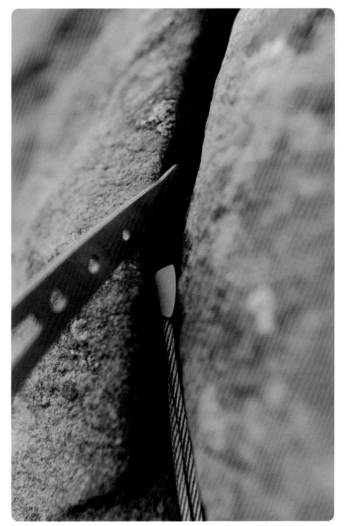

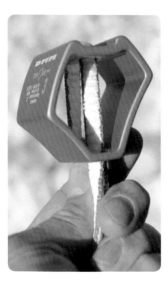

← **A DMM Torque nut, size 3. Hex-shaped nuts are very useful and, thanks to their irregular faces, they can be used in both tapered cracks and parallel-sided cracks.**

→ **This placement is not entirely parallel-sided, but it does illustrate how a load on the nut will force it to twist anti-clockwise. In doing so it will tighten more securely into the crack.**

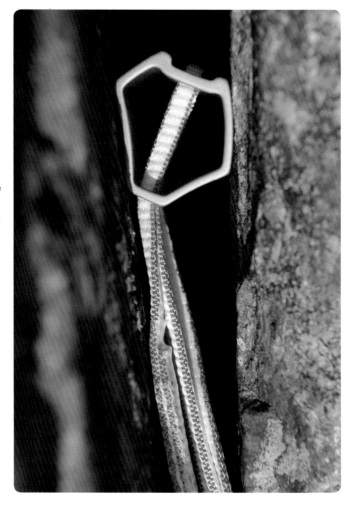

North American granite. In the days before the invention of camming devices, hexcentric nuts proved enormously effective in providing sound protection in parallel cracks.

When placed correctly, as illustrated, any load exerted on the nut will create a twisting action that tightens the nut into the placement. Unfortunately, in cracks with precisely parallel sides hexcentrics can work loose very easily and may fall out. If, however, the nut is seated with a good sharp tug this problem is largely eliminated. In fact it's rare to find perfectly parallel-sided cracks, and even a taper of a couple of degrees is enough to help seat the nut in place.

As with any nut placed on the lead, the climber must make sure that leverage on the placement is kept to an absolute minimum. Most hex-shaped nuts are threaded with a soft sling of tape and some, like those shown here, have a doubled tape that can be extended if necessary. If you think there'll be leverage on the placement despite the soft sling attachment, it can always be extended further using a quickdraw.

Hex-shaped nuts go by different names according to manufacturer and, like wedges, there's some standardisation of sizes. The range of sizes is quite broad, with the largest – and very specialised – sizes looking rather like a Swiss cowbell.

TRICAMS

These are quite a specialised item of crack protection but can be incredibly effective if placed correctly. The most likely place to use a Tricam is in solution pockets found mainly in limestone, but also occasionally in other rock types. There are climbing opportunities in many old quarries and Tricams are useful to place in drilled shot holes.

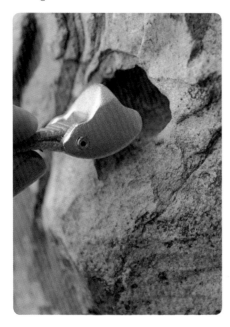

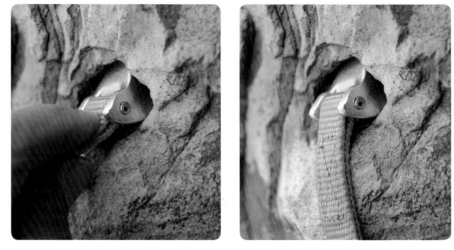

A Tricam may not have a place on every climber's rack as it's quite specialised, but it's good to have one lurking around, particularly if you trad climb on limestone where solution pockets are most often encountered. In the final photo here you can see how any load will 'cam' the nut into the pocket, creating a sound piece of protection. Always seat a Tricam with a sharp tug.

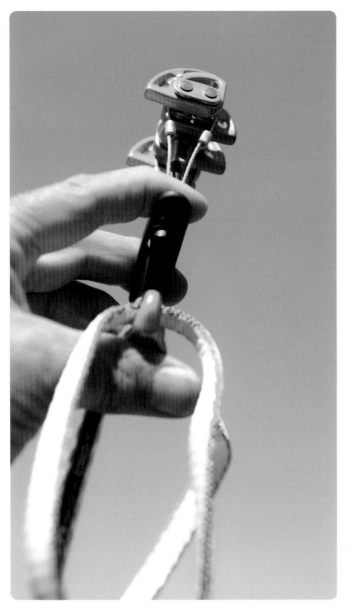

← **Prior to insertion in a crack, a cam is closed by using the thumb on the end of the stem and fingers on the trigger bar.**

CAMS

Cams are the most expensive items of climbing equipment you can buy but you could almost say they're worth their weight in gold! To kit yourself out with a full set of Black Diamond cams will cost £850 -900 at full price but they are available at discounted prices. Needless to say, very few climbers have a complete set…

Cams are the single most significant development in climbing protection over the past few decades. The principle on which they work is of individually sprung cams connected to a trigger mechanism, which is pulled to reduce the size of the cam for placement in a crack and then released so that the cam opens out and makes contact with the rock. Any load exerted on to the cams collectively should force them to open further and bite into the rock surface.

There are some essential points to note regarding the placement of cams:

■ They should never be forced tightly into a crack with the cams fully closed. Though this might give a very tight fit, they will be difficult, even impossible, to extract after being loaded.

■ The opposite is also true: cams shouldn't be placed in a crack when fully or nearly open. The cams need some leeway to expand in order to tighten within a crack and bite effectively.

■ Each of the cams should be in contact with rock so that maximum effectiveness results.

■ As a rule of thumb, the best placements are when the cams are operated within the middle third of their full travel from open to fully closed. This means that bigger cams will have a greater range of travel than smaller sizes.

Really tiny cams are highly specialised pieces of climbing equipment used for the leanest of cracks and will almost certainly be of little use when taking your first steps on rock.

As with all crack protection, cam sizes follow a numbering system, from 00 for the tiniest to 6 for the largest; some models have half sizes in between.

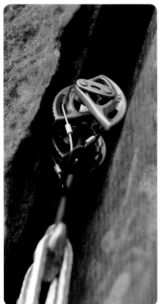

← **Perfect placing of a large cam: the cams are in the middle range of travel, neither too wide nor too tight. A cam should always be put into the crack fully closed and allowed to open once inside.**

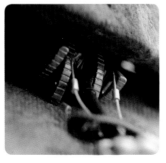

⬇ **A cam that's jammed in too tightly.**

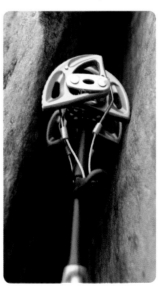

⬇ **A cam that's too open.**

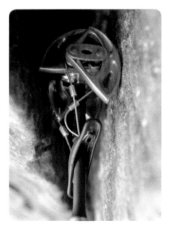

⬇ **A placement where one cam isn't biting. In desperation a climber may just stuff a cam into a crack but it usually doesn't work out too well.**

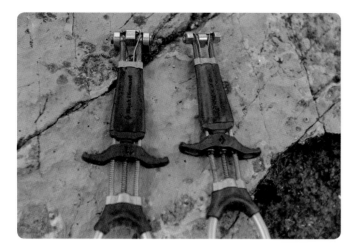

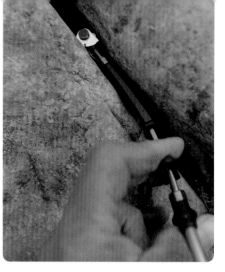

← Black Diamond C3 Camalots present a narrow profile and are useful for thin, shallow crack placements.

→ The range of cam movement is very limited with small cams.

NUTS IN OPPOSITION

Crack protection can be arranged using nuts or cams in opposition to each other. As you gain more experience, you may encounter situations where using crack protection in this way affords the only solid means of security available. A typical scenario is where you come across a horizontal crack where gear can be placed sideways, in opposition to each other.

There are several ways to arrange nuts in two placements so that the load point is central and divided reasonably equally between the two nuts.

→ **Nuts placed in opposition to each other. With the method illustrated it is vital to put the extra turn in one strand of the sling around the karabiner as shown in the second image.**

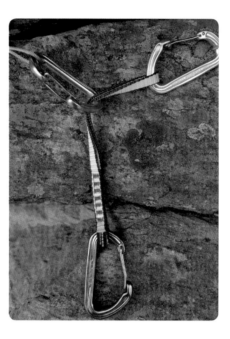

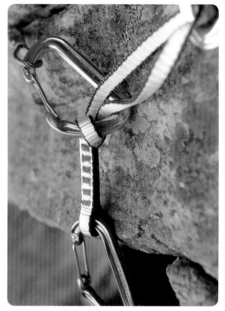

↓→ **A second method uses a single sling with a twist in one strand at the attachment point. This is a self-equalising twist that allows the load to be equally spread whatever the direction it may come from.**

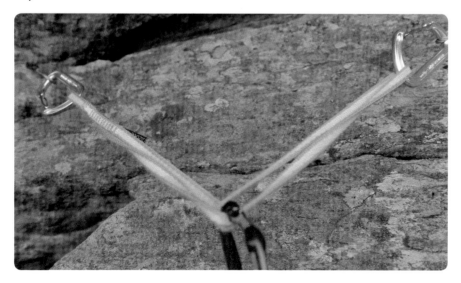

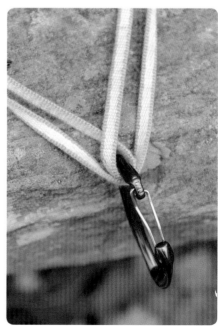

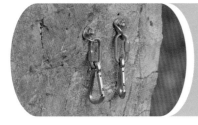

There are other ways to arrange protection to create anchors and for leader protection. Some of these rely on natural features whereas others may be placed permanently in the rock. Those that are placed permanently are usually subject to an unwritten but strictly observed code of practice.

SLINGS

Slings are used in various ways. The simplest methods are around trees or chockstones (rocks or boulders jammed across a crack or chimney). In some rock types, such as limestone, small but solid thread placements may be found in the rock face itself.

Trees on crags can be embraced as sound anchors if you feel that they're well rooted and living. Many climbs have trees on ledges or growing out of cracks, and climbers must show respect for them and use them considerately and with gratitude. It's not good for a tree to be repeatedly caressed by moving ropes or slings as it can wear through the bark and cause the tree's slow demise.

Slings are threaded around or through the anchor and the two end loops are clipped together using a screwgate karabiner (for an anchor) or a snaplink (for a running belay to protect the lead climber). Slings can also be used draped over a spike or flake of rock or around a large boulder on the ground.

Slings are commonly made from tape and the ends are stitched together by the manufacturer to create a closed loop. It's usual nowadays for the tape to be made from Dyneema, which is immensely strong, light and hard-wearing, but other options are nylon in pure or tubular woven forms; nylon slings can be purchased stitched but are also available off the roll for making up knotted slings.

Tape made from Dyneema is usually around 1cm in width, though narrower types are available, while nylon tape can be up to 2cm wide. Slings also come in various lengths, with the measurement determined by

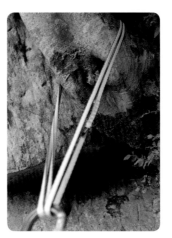

⬆ **This holly tree provides a good anchor: a long sling is placed around the tree and the end loops are clipped with a screwgate karabiner.**

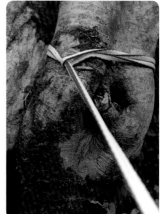

⬆ **Here the sling has been 'larksfooted' or 'girth-hitched' around the tree to negate any sliding movement.**

the total length of the tape: a 1.2m sling can be carried over the shoulder and a 2.4m sling can be carried doubled over the shoulder. Slings of 6m are available and have more specialised applications in constructing anchors by linking them together; these slings go by the technical term of cordelette.

Slings are also useful for bringing multiple anchor points together to a central fixing point (see Chapter 6).

There are some key points to remember for the safe use of slings:
- Never stretch a sling tightly around a flake or bollard of rock.
- If a sling is stretched too tight, use a larger one or even consider using the rope if the anchor is going to be used for a belay stance.

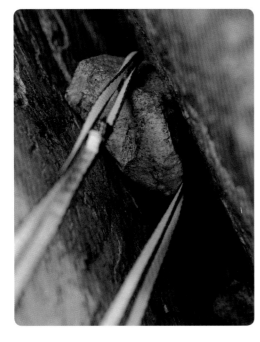

⬅ **A chockstone wedged in a crack can be threaded with a sling. Just make sure there isn't even the tiniest chink of light between the jammed rock and the sides of the crack, as the sling could pull through a small gap under load.**

⬇ **A small but comfortingly solid limestone thread. Check that there are no sharp edges that might damage the sling. Bring the loops of the threaded sling together and connect them with a karabiner.**

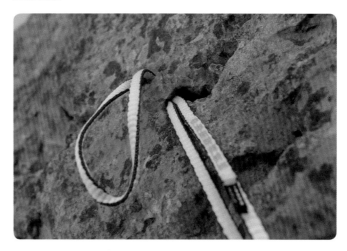

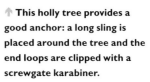

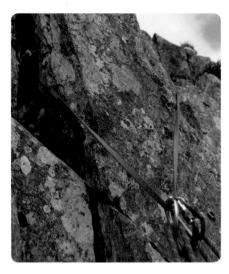

↑ A sling draped around a flake and used as an anchor. You must check that a flake is a solid part of the mountain before deciding to use it for an anchor. Even quite tiny flakes can be used for protection if they're integral features of the rock face.

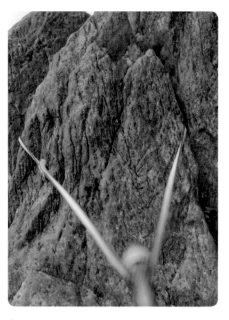

↑ This flake is well embedded into the cliff; try to get the sling around it as far down as possible.

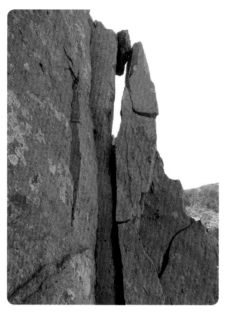

↑ This feature wouldn't be a good choice of anchor…

■ However you place a sling, the angle created when it's loaded via a karabiner should, ideally, not exceed 20–30 degrees. Angles beyond this place greater strain on the sling when it's under load and the advertised breaking strain of the sling may be exceeded once the angle reaches 120 degrees or greater.

■ Make sure that the sling isn't in contact with any sharp edges of rock. This is particularly important when threading jammed rocks in cracks. A sling under load can cut through quite easily over a sharp edge.

QUICKDRAWS

A quickdraw, sometimes called an 'extender', is normally used to extend running belays in order to reduce leverage on the placement or to avoid what's known as rope drag. Rope drag can occur when the rope is clipped into several running belays one after another. If the runners are alternately off to one side, the rope will zigzag up the cliff, causing friction – maybe enough to halt all movement!

Quickdraws can also be used to extend runners that may be tucked in underneath an overlap of rock or around a bulge. Sometimes you may need to extend running belays so far that a sling must be used in place of a quickdraw. On sport climbs quickdraws are also used to clip into bolt protection.

One of the loops through which a karabiner is clipped is usually smaller and tighter than the other and usually contains a retaining rubber loop for the karabiner. This prevents the karabiner from spinning around in the quickdraw and makes clipping in a rope

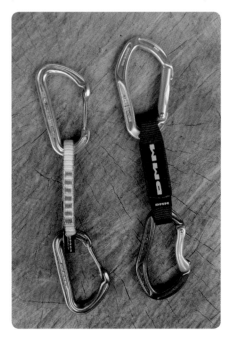

← Quickdraws are an integral part of creating good protection and are considered further in Chapter 7.

→ Slings are also used to extend running belays where a quickdraw may not be long enough; here the running belay is extended to reduce rope drag.

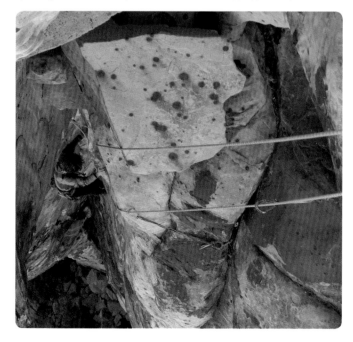

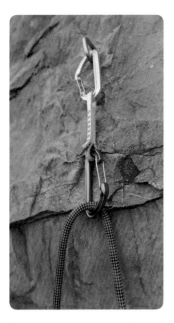

⬆ **Quickdraw arranged with karabiners facing opposite directions.**

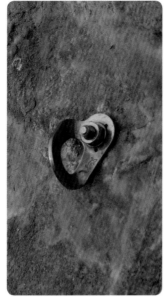

⬆ **A stainless steel through-bolt with hangar.**

⬆ **A rusted through-bolt alongside a newer resin bolt, which, of course, will be the choice to clip to.**

⬆ **A resin staple.**

considerably easier. Solid-gate karabiners usually have a curved gate to facilitate clipping in the rope.

Most quickdraws are set up so that one end is always used to clip to the piece of protection and the other is used for clipping the rope through. There is good reason for this. Karabiners clipped into wire slings on nuts and into bolts may incur damage from being clipped into metal, particularly if they are fallen on regularly. Tiny burrs, which are sometimes difficult to detect, may develop on the inside of a karabiner, and may be sharp enough to damage the climbing rope – which, of course, is your lifeline.

Different lengths of quickdraw are available, from 12cm up to around 22cm.

When setting up a quickdraw for personal use there are two options. It's important to say that there's no compelling reason why either of the methods suggested here is better than the other and so final choice will come down to personal preference through experience or from the advice of someone you respect and who has considerable climbing experience.

One way to set up the quickdraw is to have snaplink karabiner gates facing in opposite directions and the other option is with both gates facing the same way.

BOLTS

These are permanently secured anchors points on a cliff. There are several forms with the two main ones being:

- ▓ The expansion bolt (or through-bolt). Normally bolts will be 12mm in diameter but 10mm is also quite common. The bolt has a 'hangar' to which a karabiner can be clipped.
- ▓ The 'resin' or 'eco' bolt. These are placed into a drilled hole along with a hard-setting resin that, once set, secures the bolt in place. Arguably such bolts are preferable as no ingress of water can occur around the buried part of the bolt to cause undetectable damage.

Most bolts are made of carbon-manganese or alloy steel and may be

zinc-coated. Stainless steel bolts, though considerably more expensive, are preferable.

In the early days of bolting a wide variety of different types of bolt were used, some of which may still be in place more than 20 years on. It may be very difficult to determine the quality of some placements of a certain age but newer fixings are likely to be sound.

The climbers who create sport routes place the bolts and then climb the route. Placing is usually done by abseiling down the cliff and drilling with a powerful cordless drill. Occasionally, particularly on multi-pitch bolted climbs, bolts may be placed on the lead and, even more rarely, the holes for bolt placement may be made by hand.

A climb that's well bolted is exactly what it says it is – bolts at regular intervals and in places where it's relatively comfortable to hang on to a handhold with one hand and clip with the other. Climbs that are poorly bolted may have bolts spaced a long way apart, may not protect the most difficult sections of the climb adequately, and may be badly placed or of dubious quality. The worst-case scenario is where a failure to clip the second bolt up a climb could result in the climber falling to the ground. It's not uncommon to find that bolt protection becomes more widely spaced when the climbing becomes easier than the advertised grade.

An extra item of equipment used by some sport climbers is a clip stick. This is a device that allows a climber to clip bolt runners above his head, making the route considerably safer. The pole of a clip stick is extendable and some designs may reach more than 3m above you.

In the UK the placement of bolts on rock climbs or the creation of sport climbs is subject to certain limitations and unwritten rules that control where and when they can be used and what crags are most suited to sport climbing.

On single-pitch sport climbs there will be lower-off points at the top of the climb, and you will doubtless encounter several formats. In an attempt to highlight as many different styles as possible the accompanying photos show the most likely ones you'll come across – all of these styles are actually on a single sport climbing venue in the UK! The ways to use the different types of lower-off are explained in Chapter 7.

Types of lower-off

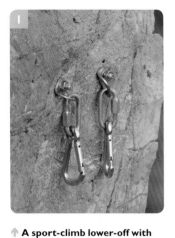

↑ **A sport-climb lower-off with easy-to-clip stainless steel karabiners.**

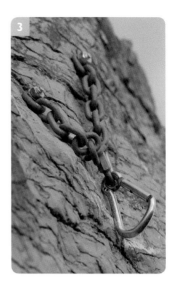

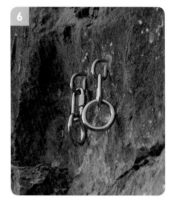

↑ **Two through-bolts with hangars and rings attached.**

➜ **Two stainless steel threaded bars with chain looped over and secured with locking nuts. The chain is brought to one central attachment point where a stainless steel snaplink karabiner is attached via a maillon for ease of clipping and lowering off.**

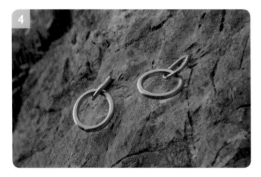

↑ **Two resin wire bolts with rings attached.**

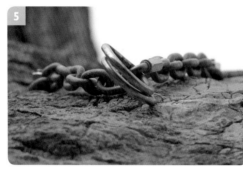

↑ **Two stainless steel threaded bars with chain looped over and secured with locking nuts. The chain is brought to one central attachment point where two stainless steel rings are attached via a maillon.**

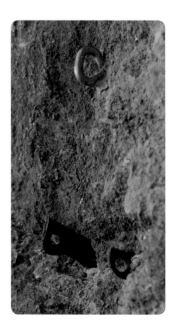

↑ **Two resin bolts with maillons and then rings attached.**

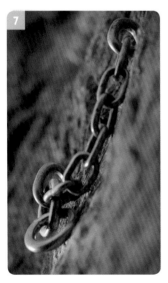

↑ **Finally the most reassuring of all – resin bolts with chain attached brought to one central point with a stainless steel ring.**

PITONS

Pitons were once used for protection on climbs where no other protection equipment could be placed. They were also often used as a 'point of aid' for a handhold or foothold to make progress, though climbers endeavour to eliminate points of aid in order to make climbs totally free. In any case the modern climber has many more options available and the use of pitons is rarely necessary, other than on aid climbs (where the ascent is impossible without pitons for direct assistance) and on winter climbs (where judicious use is common).

Very few rock climbers will come across pitons these days and even fewer will ever place one. A piton is made from mild steel or hardened steel. Mild steel pitons are designed to be put in once and left there until they rust away or work loose and fall out. The hardened steel variety may be put in and left in place but they're more suited to being removed and reused elsewhere several times.

If you do encounter pitons in situ on climbs, it can be difficult to judge their provenance and suitability. A piton that has been in place for many years should be treated with caution and it's always preferable to try to find an alternative. Corrosion can take place within the crack in which the piton has been placed and discoloration may be apparent near the surface of the rock. Pitons placed on sea cliffs rarely last very long without corrosion occurring.

↑ **Ancient pitons with a sound stainless steel resin bolt nearby.**

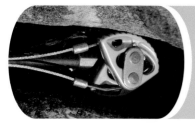

AND FINALLY...

Among the various crags where you choose to climb, you'll almost certainly come across abandoned equipment in various states of dilapidation. Such pieces, usually referred to as 'tat', may include old bits of rope or cord threaded through holes, corroded pitons or bolts, and rusting nuts wedged where no-one has managed to retrieve them.

Whenever you encounter such pieces of kit always treat them with the utmost suspicion and search for alternatives. Determining how decayed something has become may be difficult, but sun-faded slings and corroded nuts are not to be touched.

➜ **Equipment abandoned or placed by previous climbers must be treated with suspicion as it may have been there for years and be dubious safety-wise.**

⬇ **When found in situ an abseil sling or lower-off made of a variety of rope slings connected with a malingering karabiner isn't always a reassuring anchor. UV degradation of nylon occurs rapidly, and if you're unsure of the degree of UV exposure try loosening one of the knots to discover the original colour of the sling.**

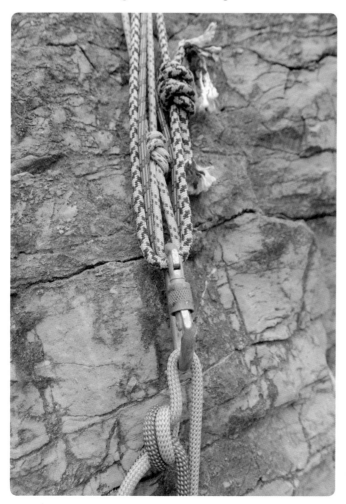

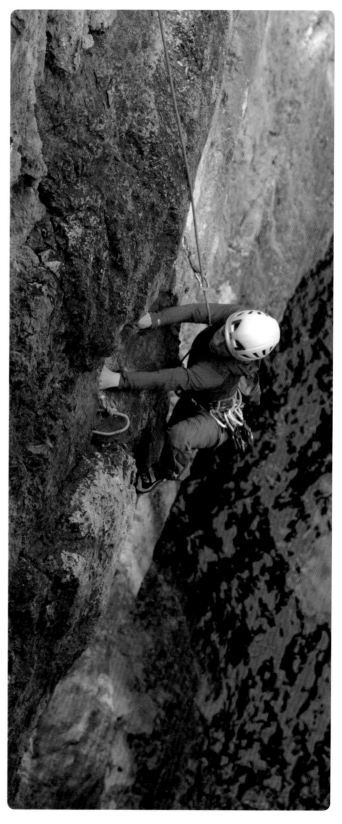

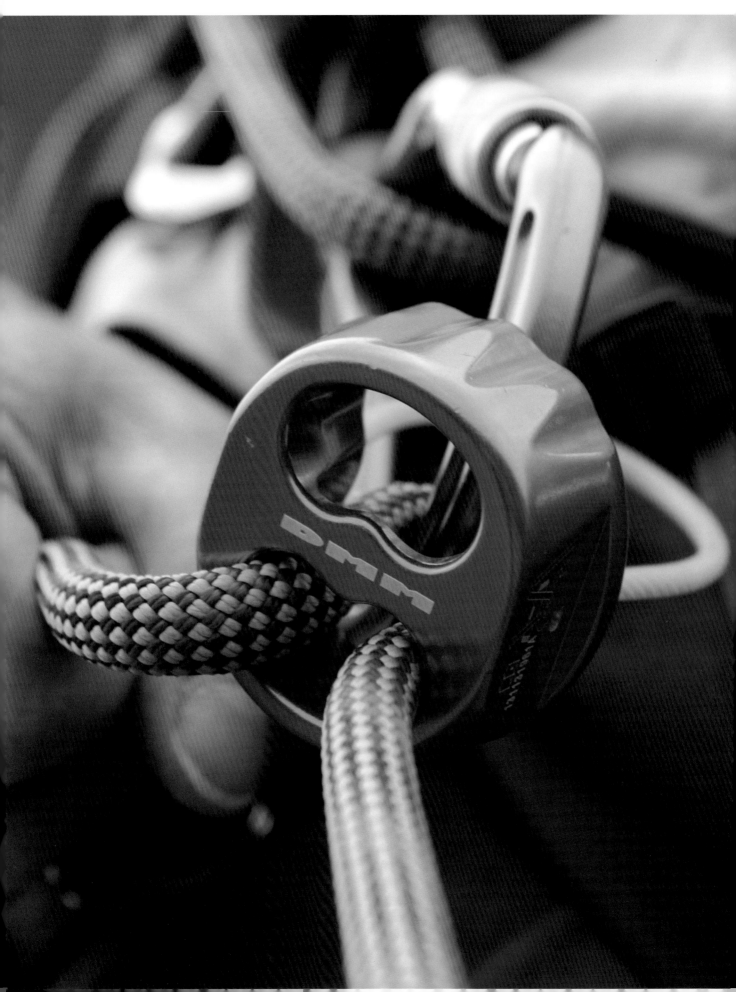

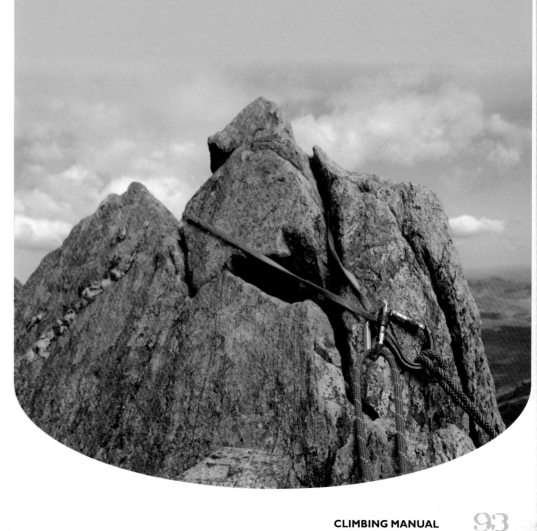

CHAPTER 6

STAYING SAFE

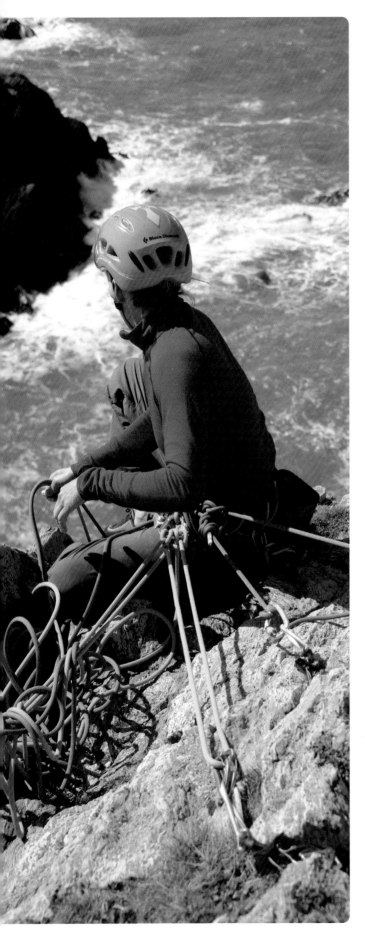

Having looked at the individual components that make up the essence of climbing safety, in this chapter we will consider some of the myriad ways in which they can all be brought together to form the complete safety chain.

Climbing safety is paramount for a long and rewarding climbing life. Misjudgement, errors and a sloppy approach to safety carry the ultimate penalty in many climbing situations. To climb safely the climber must consider many and varying factors dependent on the style of climbing. One would imagine that indoor climbing carries little risk but poor implementation of basic techniques has led to accidents and severe injury. Top roping, bottom roping and sport climbing are all generally considered safe activities, but things can and do go wrong, and climbers get injured due to carelessness or a poor attitude towards safety. Trad climbing has the highest risk of all climbing styles (except for soloing, where no safety equipment is used) and the components of the safety chain may be considered the most complex.

When learning, it's best to have close supervision from an experienced companion or a professionally qualified instructor or mountain guide. Under their tutelage you can be assured that safety is never compromised and the wealth of knowledge that you will glean will stand you in good stead for future climbing adventures.

Consider safety in all its forms as of fundamental importance and remember that it isn't only an individual responsibility but also a team effort when companions are involved.

← **Arranging anchors at the top of a climb or on a ledge part way up is a complex but vital part of the whole safety chain. It requires much practice and good judgement to create a sound anchor and attach yourself to it. Here the leader is attached to four anchors at the top of a sea cliff.**

⬇ **An anchor rigged for bottom roping. In this case the anchors are already in place by means of fixed rings and cables, but you still need to know how to connect the anchor rope safely.**

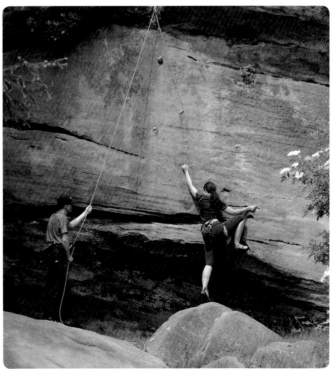

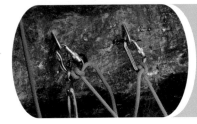

CREATING AND USING SAFE ANCHORS

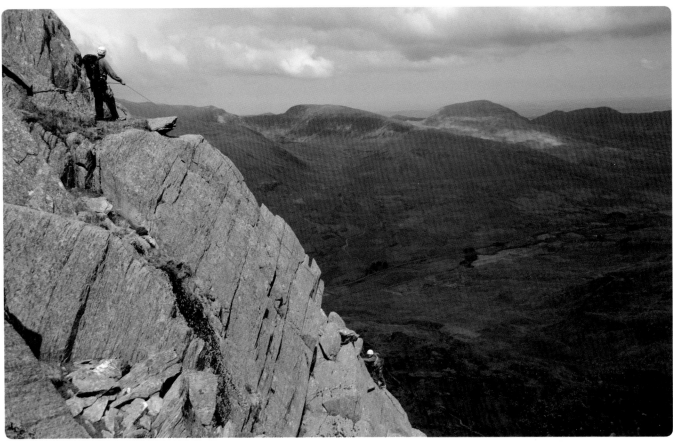

The creation of safe anchors is the essence of all climbing safety. All of the principles discussed in this section can be applied to the various climbing situations in which you will need a sound anchor. Here are a few:

- Bottom roping: arranging an anchor at the top of a single-pitch climb so that climbers can be safeguarded on routes by the rope held by a belayer standing on the ground.
- Top roping: arranging an anchor at the top of a single-pitch climb so that the climber can be belayed from above.
- Arranging an anchor for abseil practice.
- Arranging an anchor for retreating from a climb.
- Making secure anchors at the end of a pitch of climbing on multi-pitch climbs.
- Creating an anchor to take an upward pulling force to prevent a belayer being pulled upwards in the event of having to hold a fall by the leader.
- Making yourself secure at the start of a climb that's situated above threatening terrain.

As a basic principle, any anchor you create should be strong enough to hold any force that might be exerted upon it. These forces will vary according to a particular situation: in some instances forces could be relatively low, in others extremely powerful. Though this might suggest

⬆ **A large block on a ledge might provide a sound anchor but it needs to weigh several tons to be truly sound.**

that there could be different levels of security when creating anchors, in reality anchors must always be able to sustain the most severe loads imaginable. Using this premise, safety is always assured.

TYPES OF ANCHOR

We've already considered the basics of anchor creation in the previous chapter. Now we need to look at the types of anchor and then the methods that can be used to attach ourselves to them.

The simplest anchor and possibly the one that inspires the most confidence is a large, deeply rooted tree. Provided that it's possible to get a sling around the main trunk, such anchors are simple to rig and one tree anchor will suffice.

The next simplest is perhaps a large flake of rock that stands proud from a rock face or ledge. If the flake is part of the rock face, check to see that it's well attached and not just perched precariously on a ledge. A good way to test for solidity is to tap it lightly with a screwgate karabiner. Any hollowness to the sound means that it isn't attached, whereas a non-reverberating, dull sound usually means that it's part of the rock face. An extremely large flake or boulder sitting on a ledge can also provide a simple and sound anchor, but, of

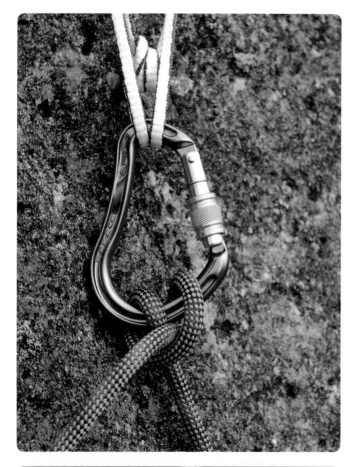

← Whenever you secure yourself to anchor points or safeguard a climbing partner using a belay device, always use a screwgate karabiner with the locking sleeve securely tightened. Ensure that the karabiner is appropriate for the task. Round-ended karabiners are essential for clipping several knots to the same karabiner and for use with belaying devices.

course, the weight of the flake or boulder is important. Something that looks like it weighs a good tonne or so should prove to be stable, but something that can be moved or lifted even the tiniest amount is most definitely not.

A rock or small boulder wedged in a wide crack may also provide a suitable anchor. These are called chockstones and there's often a gap around which a sling can be threaded and the two ends joined using a screwgate karabiner. Again, provided that you can get a sling around the feature, in many cases a single anchor may suffice. A sling threaded around an anchor in this way is termed by climbers as a 'thread' for short.

Whenever you use a sling to create a rock anchor it's vital to check that there are no sharp edges over which it might run. Even a small, ragged edge to the rock can damage a sling, particularly when it's loaded.

When it comes to using crack protection devices to create anchors, life becomes a little more complex.

There are very few situations in climbing where one will rely solely on a single nut or cam placed in a crack as an anchor, no matter how sound the placement, so the suggested rule is a minimum of two. One exception to this, however, is when placing running belays on the lead to protect the lead climber (see Chapter 7).

If a single anchor point were to fail under extreme load there would be no back-up. Two anchor placements not only provide back-up but they can be arranged so that any load is divided equally between them; in some instances one might use a third, fourth or even a fifth anchor.

ATTACHING TO ANCHORS

In general try to use screwgate karabiners to attach to anchor points. If necessary snaplinks can be used but make sure that the rope or sling cannot detach itself accidentally. If you're obliged to use a snaplink, a good rule to follow is to ensure that the attachment is out of arm's reach and will remain constantly under some tension. As an alternative to screwgates, it's possible to utilise two snaplink krabs with gates facing in opposite directions.

There are various methods of linking anchors together using slings to form one central point of attachment. The advantage of a single point of attachment is that it's much less complicated to use when belaying your partner or rigging anchor points at the top of a single-pitch crag venue for top or bottom roping. Regardless of the method used, the most important message to get across is that the failure of one anchor shouldn't cause any shock loading on the remaining anchor or anchors.

Here are three suggested ways to use a sling to form a single point of attachment:

■ Clip the sling into a screwgate karabiner on each anchor. Find the direction from which you anticipate any loading will come and tie

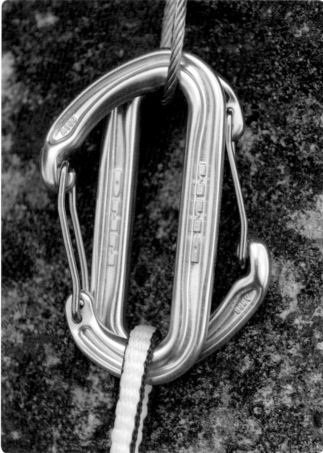

← If you find yourself short of screwgate karabiners, two snaplinks arranged 'back to back' are a very good alternative.

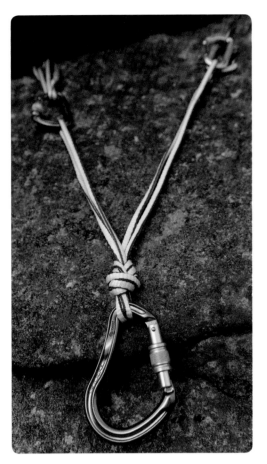

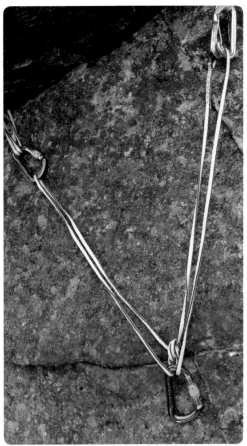

←← **Two anchor points brought together to form a single attachment point. Use a figure of eight knot or an overhand. Both are acceptable.**

← **A second method of bringing two anchors together using a sling: the overhand knot is tied after clipping in to one anchor point and adjusted after clipping into the second. The principle of loading each anchor equally must always be followed.**

an overhand knot in the doubled sling. The loop created by tying the overhand is where you attach any ropes or climbers.

■ Clip one end of the sling into one of the anchors. Tie an overhand knot at the mid-point of the sling and then clip the other end into the second anchor. Decide which direction any loading will come from and move the overhand knot along the sling until you effectively create two 'separate' slings that are under equal tension when loaded. The attachment point to the anchor is then through the two sling loops.

■ The third method is handy but only applicable in situations where you're certain that the anchors are solid and where you may have to change your position on the stance to accommodate loading from several different directions. This method is known as a 'sliding equal' or 'rolling X'.

One further method of forming a single point of attachment involves the use of a cordelette – a long sling typically 4m in length. Cordelettes can be tricky to carry as there's so much tape to bundle up and attach to the harness, but they're invaluable for bringing multiple anchors together to one central point.

Finally, it's important to discuss angles. When you use a sling to connect two anchors together as illustrated here, the angle created in the sling at the attachment point has a significant bearing on how the loading is distributed between both anchors. At an angle of 20 degrees or less, the load

will be divided equally between both anchors. Angles greater than 20 degrees increase the loading incrementally on each anchor, and at 120 degrees each anchor will take the full load. If you're concerned that angles will reach a critical point, it's better to use a longer sling, such as a cordelette, or a different method of attachment.

↓ **The cordelette is a very useful sling to clip several anchors together though quite awkward to bundle up to carry. After clipping in to each anchor point and equalising the sling, tie an overhand knot to form the attachment loop.**

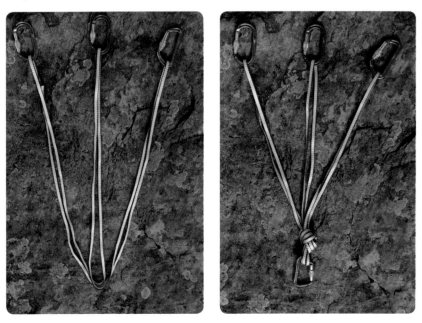

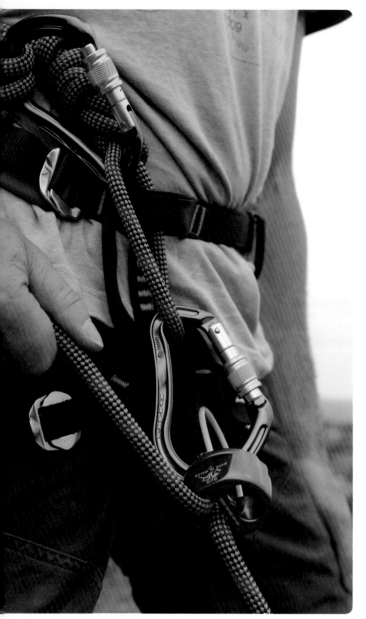

← When you need to attach yourself to an anchor point, it's important to clip through the rope loop that's formed when you tie in to the end of rope; the belay device is attached to the same point. If the rope to your anchor is tight, some of the strain of holding a climber can be transferred on to the anchor, not directly on to the belayer.

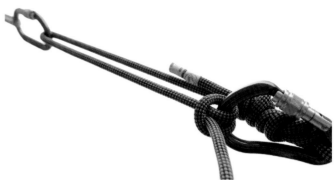

↑ Using the rope, clip through a screwgate karabiner on the anchor point and secure to the rope tie-in loop using a clove hitch.

↓ If your single anchor point is within comfortable arm's reach, it's possible to secure yourself directly to it with a clove hitch.

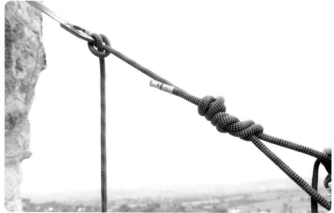

USING THE CLIMBING ROPE TO ATTACH TO ANCHORS

There are a few situations where climbers will use the rope to attach directly to anchor points: on a stance part way up a multi-pitch climb; at the top of a climb; and at the start of a climb in situations where you're not secure while standing or sitting on the ground.

In these situations you would ideally bring anchors together to one central point and tie securely using the climbing rope. There are more than a few methods of doing this but to begin with it's better to focus on those that are simplest and most adaptable, as follows:

◼ Take the climbing rope from the tie-in point to the harness up to the anchor screwgate karabiner, clip it in and screw the locking sleeve shut. The rope can then be secured back to the harness using a clove hitch attached to the central tie-in loop via a screwgate karabiner. Tighten the clove hitch, making sure that the rope back to the anchor has some tension in it and you can lean against that tension to gain support from the anchor if required. It's

possible to make the tie back to the harness using a figure of eight on the bight, but this makes it more difficult to gauge the correct tension.

◼ Clip the rope directly to the anchor point. This method can only be used effectively when there's a single point to attach to and that single point is comfortably within an arm's reach of where you will stand or sit to belay. It's possible to use this method out of arm's reach, but it's less easy to adjust tension in the anchor to the ideal.

→ Occasionally it may be sensible to clip to an anchor using a sling with some slack in it, such as on a large but exposed ledge at the start of a climb over steep ground or above the sea. Having a small amount of slack means that you can move around a little if needed. It's important that this is put in context with the overall safety chain and such anchor attachments are intended to hold body weight only – not severe loads.

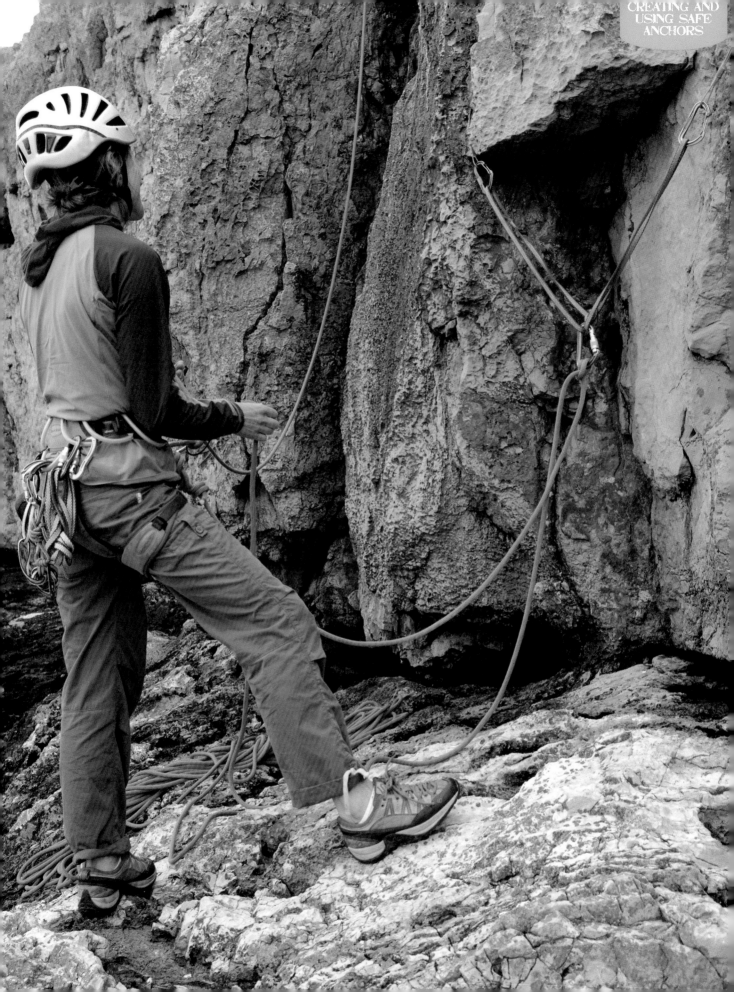

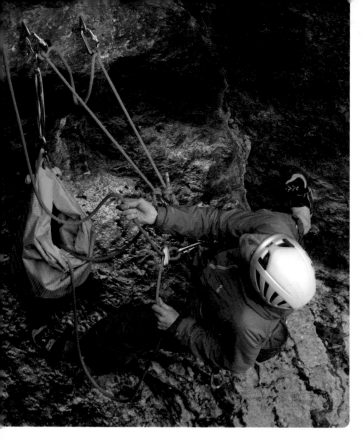

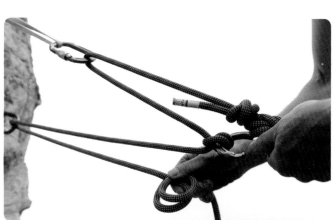

↑ **Using the rope to secure to two anchors with clove hitches. It's vitally important to use a large, round-ended HMS karabiner when clipping in two or more clove hitches to the same krab.**

← **Here the belayer is on a 'hanging stance' above the sea and there are two fixed stainless steel resin bolt anchors. The climbing rope is clipped directly into one, there's a small loop of slack between it and the second clip, and finally that's secured back to an HMS karabiner into the tie-in rope loop.**

▪ If you have two anchor points that are too far apart to connect together with the sling (using one of the methods illustrated in the previous section), a single climbing rope can be used. Clip the rope into one anchor, taking it back to the harness and securing it using a clove hitch, and then simply repeat the process for the second anchor. The karabiner on the central loop of the harness tie-in must be a large, pear-shaped (HMS) type in order to accommodate two clove hitches tied side by side.

▪ Another method utilises two anchors linked together to a single attachment by means of a sling, with a third anchor closer to where the belayer will sit or stand. This serves two main purposes: to prevent any rope stretch creating slack in the anchor tie-in; and, of course, to provide a third anchor point. Situations where this might be needed are commonly found at the top of a climb where the main anchors are a long way back from the edge of the cliff.

▪ It's also possible to clip directly to an anchor using a sling. This is most useful when you're belaying at the foot of a climb, particularly at an indoor wall when you might need to attach to an upward-pulling anchor where there's a weight imbalance between you and your climbing partner. It's also useful for attaching to an anchor at the start of a climb where there's a degree of risk that you might fall over an edge.

▪ One final suggestion – the rethreaded figure of eight on the bight – is handy if you should find yourself in the unlikely situation of having run out of suitable screwgate karabiners to secure clove hitches

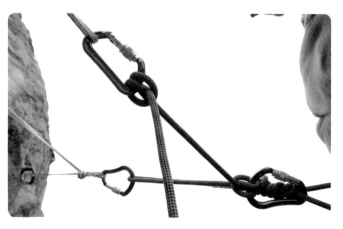

↑ **Two anchors are brought to a central attachment point using a sling. The climbing rope is clipped through a screwgate karabiner and secured back at the harness tie-in loop with a clove hitch. The second anchor attachment is within comfortable arm's reach of the belayer and can be clipped directly using a clove hitch.**

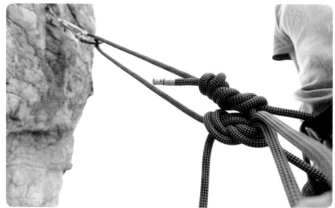

↑ **If you should run out of suitable karabiners, you can secure yourself with a rethreaded figure of eight on the bight. Make sure that you leave a long tail for safety. Several anchors could be connected in this way, the only limitations being availability of rope and the number of knots you can get into the tie-in rope loop.**

back to the harness. This method assumes that you'll also have a reasonable amount of rope available to tie the knot or, with more than one anchor, knots.

As mentioned already in Chapter 4, after tying a knot it's vital to ensure that there's sufficient tail end remaining so that security is assured.

USING A STATIC ROPE TO BRING SEVERAL ANCHORS TOGETHER

Adaptations of the methods described above can be used for rigging anchors for single-pitch climbing where the belaying is done from below (bottom roping) or for rigging a practice abseil. The same principles of loading apply: always rig so that load is divided equally between anchors.

➡ **Always attach the climbing rope through a screwgate karabiner. Here two karabiners are used to reduce the friction on the rope by creating a wider curve for it to pass round.**

⬇ **This is a suggested method for bringing several anchors to one central tie-in point when arranging a bottom rope for single-pitch climbing. Some of the anchors themselves can be linked with a sling, as shown previously, and the static climbing rope secured with a screwgate karabiner. Static or non-stretch ropes are useful for these situations as there's very little movement across the rock when taking the weight of a climber.**

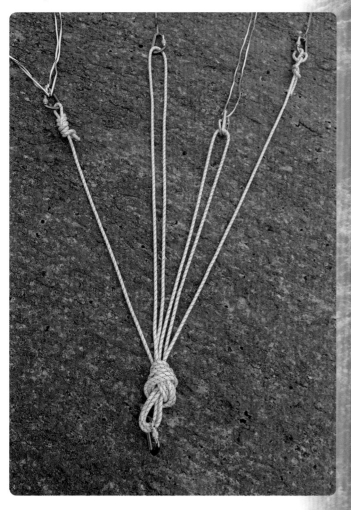

BELAY DEVICES

When climbers safeguard each other using a rope it's called belaying. The various ways to belay a climber include using body belays where the rope is wrapped around the waist or shoulder, or using knots that can be attached via a screwgate karabiner directly to an anchor. In this section, however, we will concentrate on methods that are far more secure, using specific devices designed for the task.

For simplicity, belay devices can be broadly categorised into two types:

Slotted belay devices These are the most common and also less sophisticated. Most devices feature two slots, enabling the climber to use the same device for both single-rope technique and double-rope technique (see Chapter 7). Additionally, double-slotted devices can be used for abseiling down single or double ropes (see Chapter 8). Most slotted devices will accommodate rope diameters from 8.8mm to 11mm; rope diameters less than 8.8mm require smaller slots for effective braking of the rope.

Mechanical belay devices Here there are fewer choices available and those that come into this category tend to be much more specialised.

Belay devices work by creating friction between rope and device in order to assist the belayer in holding a fallen climber, be they a second or a leader. In order to do this efficiently, it's necessary to create more friction by angling the slack rope over the rim of the device to create a sharp 'S' bend in the rope.

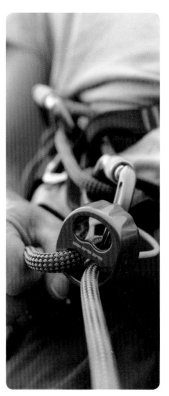

Operating a belay device requires a rigid skill base for safety. Whether you're safeguarding a climber from above or below, and regardless of the type of device used, you must never completely let go of the controlling rope. If you do and at that very moment the climber falls, you'll never regain control of the rope to stop their fall. In this photo the right hand holds the controlling rope and the left holds the rope going directly to the climber.

A belay device held in a locked-off position when belaying a climber from above.

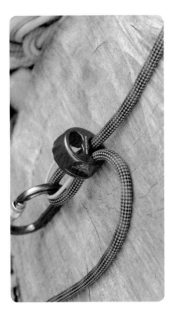
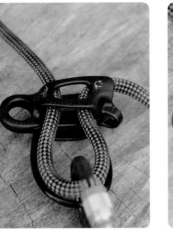
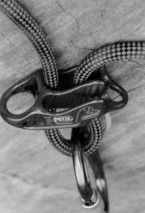
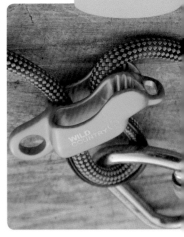

Four slotted belay devices, left to right: DMM BUG, Black Diamond ATC (Air Traffic Controller) Pro, Petzl Reverso 4, Wild Country Pro Guide. The latter three devices are suited for use as a direct belay, which is covered in Chapter 9.

If the reaction of the belayer in arresting a fall is fast and immediate, the fall can be halted very suddenly and with great effect. However, circumstances conspire to make this almost impossible and the arresting of a fall in practice tends to be more gradual, taking one or two seconds when the belayer is alert to the situation. This is a good thing and is referred to as a dynamic belay. The advantage is mainly that the load is absorbed gradually as each part of the safety chain comes into effect and ultimately puts much less strain on the system.

By contrast, if climbers were to use relatively rigid, non-stretch ropes and belay devices that locked solid immediately they were loaded, the system of anchors and leader protection would be subjected to a force far greater and more shocking than is desirable; in some circumstances this might be enough for kit to fail.

Prior to the invention and adoption of belay devices, during the late 1960s and early 1970s, climbers would use methods of wrapping the rope around the body (waist or shoulders) to create the friction necessary to hold a fall. This was always much more insecure and unreliable, and, in conjunction with a lack of sophisticated protection equipment, gave rise to the saying that 'a leader should never fall'.

One overriding safety principle applies to correct operation of any belay device – the belayer must *never* release his grip on the essential controlling rope.

SLOTTED BELAY DEVICES

DMM Bug, Black Diamond ATC Guide, Petzl Reverso 4 and Wild Country Pro Guide – these are four examples of the double-slotted variety of belay device. The latter two devices can also be used in more specialised applications that are mostly used by climbing instructors and mountain guides.

With the exception of the Bug, each of the above-named devices – and others like them – utilises a notched slot over which the controlling or 'never let go' rope runs, and this provides the full braking effect when holding a falling climber. Though the Bug doesn't feature the notched slot, it remains a very smooth device to use due to the wide-radius curvature of its lock-over rim. All these types of belay device double up as an abseil device (see Chapter 8).

The Click Up belay device, introduced in 2013, is a relative newcomer to the climbing safety scene. The single-rope version is shown here but a double-rope version, called the Alpine Up, is also available. It doesn't really fit comfortably into either category of belay device as it's something of a super-efficient 'best of both worlds'. The Click Up is an excellent belay device to use when starting out as it functions in a simple but highly effectively way: taking in and paying out the rope is smooth and, most significantly, it has a semi-automatic locking mode when the belayer needs to hold a falling climber; an added advantage is that it comes with its own locking HMS karabiner. It's important to use rope of the recommended diameter (8.9–10.5mm) with this device; thinner ropes aren't secured effectively and thicker ropes are awkward to take in and pay out.

↓ **The Click Up.**

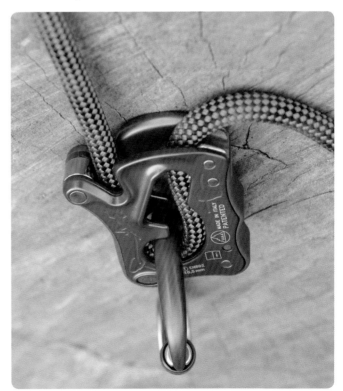

MECHANICAL BELAY DEVICES

The Petzl GriGri is the best such devices. It works on the principle of a locking cam that grips the rope when it's put under tension and can be released – by opening the cam using a lever – when a climber needs to be lowered. The device will lock automatically when a sudden load is placed on the rope, but this doesn't mean that you can let go of the controlling rope entirely. The GriGri is intended for use only on single-rope, single-pitch climbs at an indoor wall or outdoor sports climbing venue.

The GriGri is tricky to use when paying out rope in haste to a lead climber as it has a tendency to lock up when rope is pulled through quickly. This is usually most unhelpful to a leader desperate to clip a piece of protection. To operate the device effectively you need a certain amount of dexterity and practice, and you must keep a hand continually on the controlling rope.

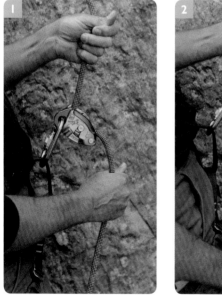

⬆ **A mechanical belay device: the Petzl GriGri.**

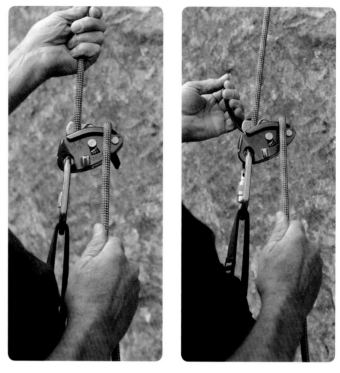

⬆ **When lowering a climber with the GriGri, the controlling rope is passed over the curled edge while the other hand releases the locking mechanism by means of a lever, which must be pulled back only far enough for the rope to begin to slide; if you pull the lever all the way back there's very little friction and the rope slides through the device with alarming speed.**

Avoiding inadvertent lock-up with a GriGri

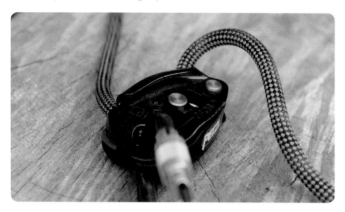

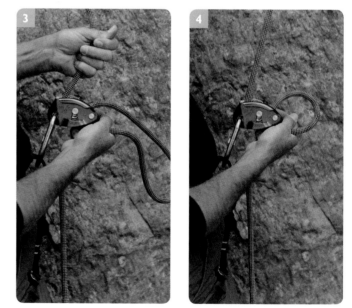

⬆ **Even though the GriGri is a semi-automatic locking belaying device, it's vital to keep hold of the controlling rope. When rope is paid out to a leader, the GriGri doesn't always differentiate between a falling climber and rapid paying-out of the rope, and tends to lock up. These photos show a suggested sequence to help to avoid inadvertent lock-up while still maintaining a grip on the controlling rope.**

⬆ **Slide the controlling hand down the rope and grip it lightly. Bring the hand back up to the device and rest it on the cam lever while pulling the rope through with the other hand. Repeat for more rope. This technique only needs to be used when paying out rope so that the leader can clip a running belay. At all other times pushing the rope through with the controlling hand and pulling with the other is normally smooth enough.**

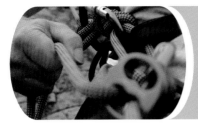

USING A BELAY DEVICE IN DIFFERENT SITUATIONS

Rock climbers use belay devices in various climbing scenarios. Many can be used to safeguard the climber in all situations, some are better for particular applications, and there are those that are wholly unsuited for anything but a specific purpose.

BOTTOM ROPING

The belay device will be used for taking in the rope as the climber ascends and for lowering the climber back to the ground. The main applications are at single-pitch venues and at indoor climbing walls.

When practising use of the belay device for the first few times, it's a good idea to have a back-up belayer to hold the slack rope just in case you inadvertently let go of the control rope at a critical point.

The belayer needs to decide whether it will be more comfortable to sit or to stand. Standing is preferable as this allows greater variance in your control of the rope.

⬇ **When you use a belay device for the first few times, it's a good idea to have a safety back-up belayer. In this photo an instructor supervises a belayer and a back-up belayer. The climber is being lowered and must keep weight on the rope at all times. It's about trusting your belayer…**

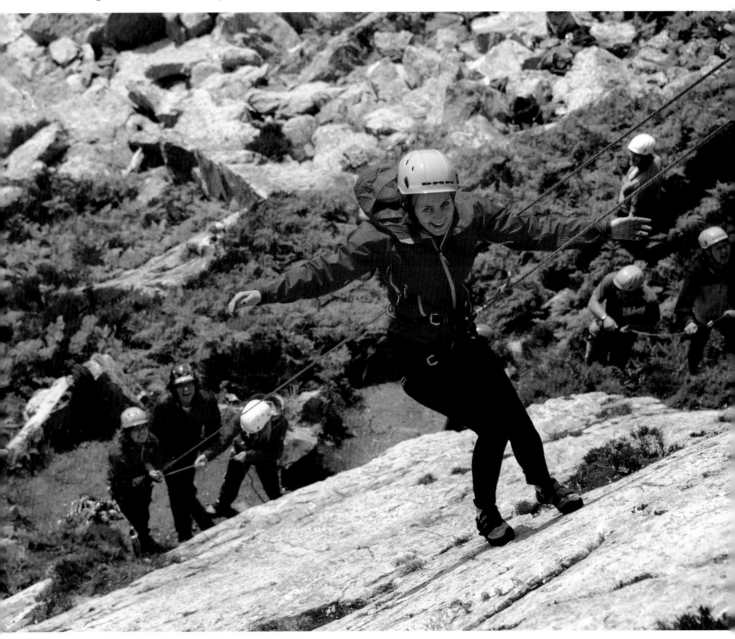

Procedure for taking in

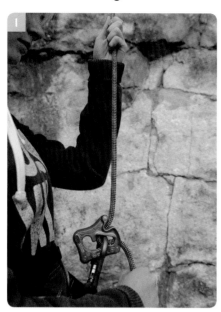

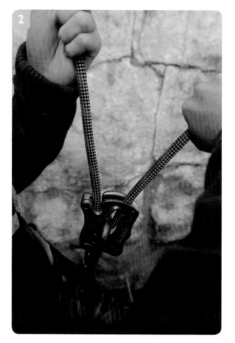

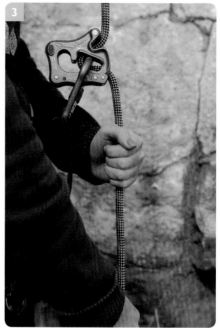

⬆ The starting position for the taking-in process when belaying for bottom roping, with the right hand holding the controlling rope. This sequence shows use of a **Click Up** but applies to all belay devices.

⬆ Point the device in the direction from which the rope is coming, pull through with the controlling hand and push through with the other.

⬆ Take the rope into the locked position and bring the left hand down to hold the controlling rope.

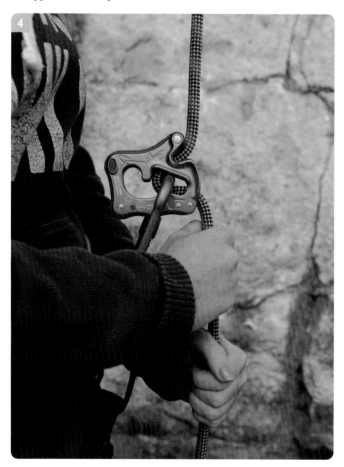

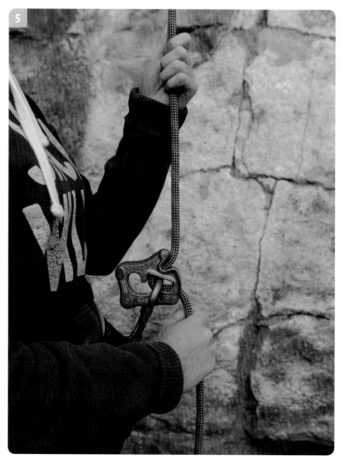

⬆ Move the right hand up to a position between the belay device and the left hand.

⬆ Return to the starting position and repeat the process. In this way you'll never let go of the controlling rope. It requires a good deal of practice.

When taking in the rope you must ensure that you retain a grip that you will lock off if you need to hold the climber's weight. There's a standard procedure for taking in (illustrated in the accompanying photo sequence) that applies to all belay devices regardless of type or style.

It's also important to consider the difference, if significant, in the weight of the climber and the weight of the belayer. A small person weighing say 40kg will have little chance of holding an 80kg climber effectively. The belayer will almost certainly be lifted off the ground should they need to hold a fall or to lower the climber.

To counter the weight imbalance, the belayer may need to be anchored to the ground using an upward-pulling anchor, so that part of the load can be shared with the anchor. At indoor climbing venues suitable anchors are often provided in the form of a sandbag to which a belayer attaches. At an outdoor single-pitch venue anchors need to be arranged with whatever is available – a tree, nuts or cams in cracks, or even a thread or sling anchor on a boulder.

The most important thing to remember from a safety point of view is that the anchoring rope to the climber should remain under a moderate amount of tension at all times. This is particularly important when the climber is within the first few metres of the ground, when the stretch in the rope could cause the climber to hit the ground as a result of a fall.

If the climber has difficulty on a section of the climb, get the rope as tight as possible by stepping away from the crag a little; this may be sufficient encouragement for the climber to make the required moves. It's even possible to haul the climber up over a difficult section of climbing, but he will need to make some attempt to climb in order for this to be effective.

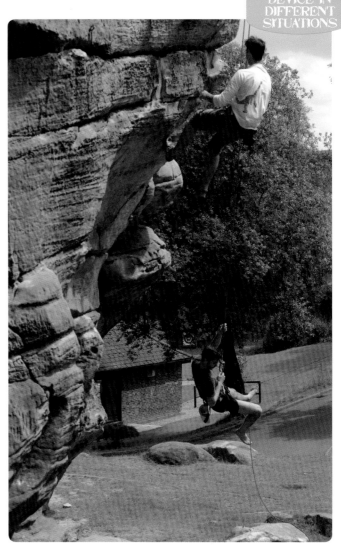

⬆ Consider any weight imbalance between the climber and the belayer. If the belayer is lighter, he or she must be attached to an upward-pulling anchor. Here the belayer has been lifted off the ground and is swinging in mid-air. He's using a standard slotted belay device and fortunately is very experienced, so he didn't let go of the controlling rope. But this situation is far from ideal.

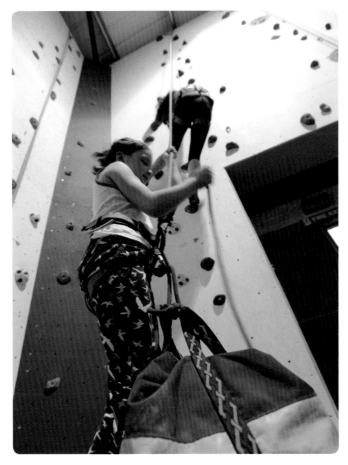

⬆ This belayer is attached to a weighty sandbag at an indoor climbing wall.

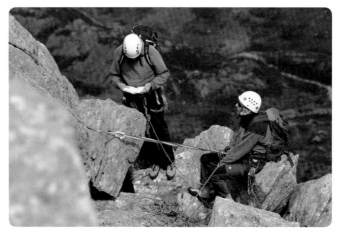

⬆ A belayer clipped to an upward-pulling anchor on the ground; this anchor is a solid 'thread' between two large rocks.

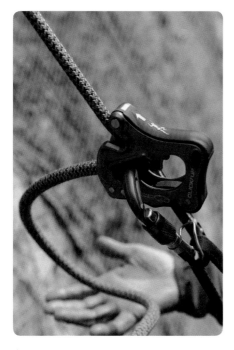

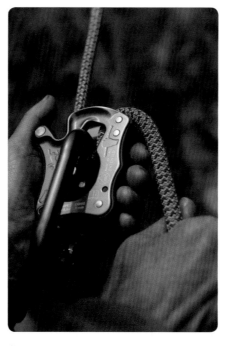

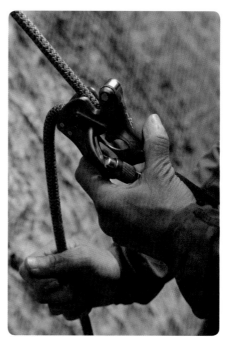

↑ When a climber reaches the top of the climb having been belayed from below, he needs to be lowered back down. The Click Up will lock when a load is placed on the rope to the climber. It's illustrated here, but letting go of the controlling rope in this way is not recommended.

↑ There are two ways to lower with the Click Up. The one illustrated in this photo is preferable as the grip on the device is more secure. The controlling rope is held in the right hand and runs across the grooved top edge. The left hand levers the device in and through the belay karabiner. The amount it is levered will determine the speed at which the rope runs.

↑ If there's a good deal of friction, or the climber being lowered is very light, it may be more comfortable to hold the Click Up as illustrated. Whichever method you use, make sure that the controlling rope runs squarely over the groove otherwise twists in the rope tend to develop.

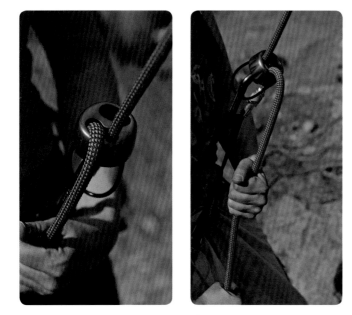

↑ Lowering with a slotted belay device. Lock the device off and use two hands on the controlling rope. It's a good idea to lean back a little against the lowering rope to keep tension on it. Simply push the rope through the device rather than let it slide through your hands. The left photo shows an incorrect method, with the controlling rope running through the device with a twist; this will work in terms of gripping power but it's better to have the control rope coming out on the side of the device that faces away from the belayer in the right-hand image.

When the time comes to lower the climber back to the ground, the belayer should take the rope as tight as possible before commencing. This will allow the climber to get comfortably tight on the rope prior to lowering and is good for confidence in the early stages. Even a half-metre of slack in the rope will mean a short 'fall' before the weight is taken. The necessary tension on the rope is best applied by taking in as tightly as possible and then stepping back from the belaying position to increase the tension. Stepping back may not be an option in some outdoor situations so the rope has to be taken as tight as possible by just pulling it through the belay device. Communication between climber and belayer is critical – never lower until both are agreed that they're prepared.

Another top tip for efficient lowering is to watch the descending climber to gauge the correct speed of descent. A comfortable speed of descent can be more easily achieved this way than keeping your eyes focussed on the belay device. You will also be able to predict when you might need to vary the speed of descent if the climber being lowered needs to step around an obstacle.

TOP ROPING

In this situation the climber is belayed from above. It is applicable to multi-pitch climbs where the leader brings up the second climber and also at single-pitch top-roping venues where the climber is belayed from above. It differs slightly from bottom roping in that it's less straightforward to give tension on the rope if it's needed and it isn't always possible to arrange an ideal place to position yourself. At the top of the climb the belayer will be anchored to the rock using methods described previously in this chapter and they will either sit or stand to belay.

When you belay a climber from above, it's generally preferable to sit or at least lean against the rock so that your position is more stable, reducing the possibility that you will be pulled aside in the event of a sudden loading of the climber's rope. However, sitting does have drawbacks. The main drawback is that it isn't so easy to give a tight rope to a climber who requests it; when standing, the belayer is also able to use some force with his legs to squat down, take the rope tightly, and then try to straighten the legs to assist with tension in the rope. In addition, another benefit of standing is that belaying a climber from above is always easier if you can see what's happening below; communication is more straightforward and the belayer can also keep a sharper eye on the climber and predict when assistance may be required or offer it when asked. As the ideal belaying position may not be possible in all scenarios, it's best to be adaptable.

The attachment to anchor points must always be in a direct line with the anticipated direction of pull if the belayer needs to take the weight of the climber. When you set up the belay, do a quick check by tracing an imaginary line from the anchor points, through the belay device and down to the climber. If any part of this line is slightly crooked, the force of a load could pull the belayer to one side. If the pull is sudden and quite forceful, sideways movement could be significant and might result in the belayer accidentally letting go of the rope. You must also ensure that the ropes to the anchor are tight, as any slack rope will result in the initial force of a load being taken on the belayer and eventually the anchor; this will be uncomfortable and will also place unnecessary extra strain on the anchor points.

Always set up the tie-in to the anchor points to come around the same side of your body as the hand that will operate the controlling rope.

When top roping, the protocol for taking in the rope is exactly the same as when bottom-roping – the security of the climber relies on the belayer not letting go of the controlling rope at any time.

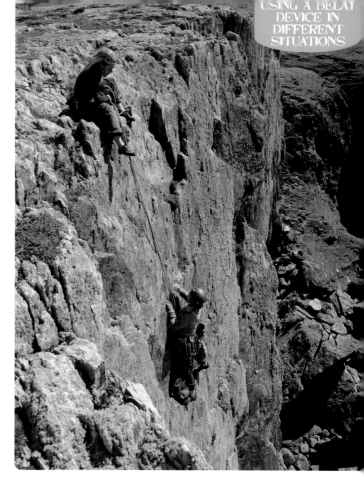

⬆ **Belaying from above, either top roping or multi-pitch, requires the same principles and rigid safety.**

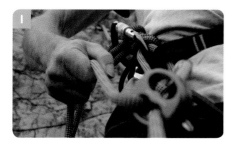

⬆ **When bringing up a climber from below, ensure that your tie-in to the anchor is tight, and also in a straight line through the harness tie-in loop directly down to the climber you are looking after.**

Procedure for top roping

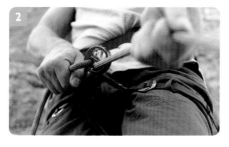

⬆ **The starting position with control rope locked off; right hand is control.**

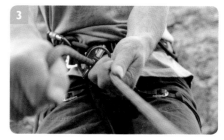

⬆ **Point the device in the direction from which the climber will arrive; pull up the rope with the left hand while pulling through with the right.**

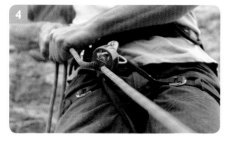

⬆ **Lock the control rope to the side and bring up the left hand to grip the rope between the device and the control hand.**

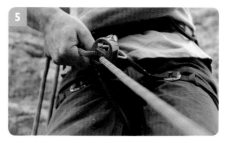

⬆ **Move the control hand to between the left hand and the device.**

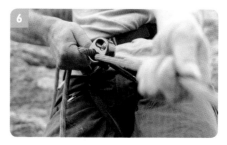

⬆ **Return to start position and repeat.**

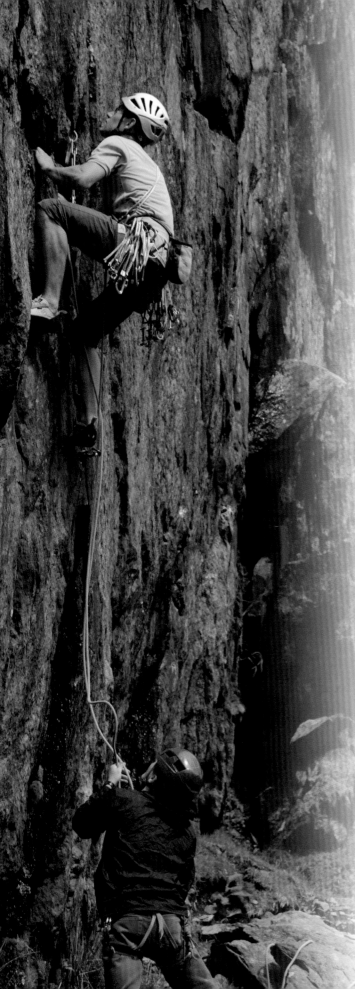

Paying out rope to a leader demands close attention and an understanding of what a leader may require. The anticipation skills needed come after a good deal of practice. In double-rope technique, it requires dexterity to pay out one rope but not the other.

BELAYING A LEADER

To belay a lead climber requires skill in handling ropes and an understanding of the different emotions a leader may go through on a particular climb. It requires careful attention and the ability and experience to predict a leader's needs at any moment on the climb. As such this is one of the most difficult and serious tasks for a climber to undertake. Quite often in climbing the most successful partnerships are built on a close understanding of how each climber in the team operates.

As a beginner it's unlikely that you'll have much understanding of what it's like to lead a climb. The stress of not having adequate or safe running belays, of finding the right line up the rock face, of fear of falling – all of these are emotional challenges a leader might experience (see Chapter 7).

The best place to learn about belaying a lead climber is on an indoor wall. While it's possible to teach yourself the basics, the techniques of belaying a leader safely are better learned under instruction and guidance from an experienced climber or a professional instructor. As always, when you first take responsibility for a new belaying scenario, it's very wise to have a second climber holding the controlling rope, 'just in case'.

There are many things to consider. The leader is totally reliant on the belayer for safety in the event of a fall so it's vital that he has total confidence in that person's ability and experience in handling a belay device. Belaying a leader carries enormous responsibility and a casual attitude will more than likely lead to accidents. Constant vigilance and attentiveness is required.

Paying out the rope is fairly straightforward. Just as with taking in the rope, it's vital that the belayer always keeps hold of the control rope with one hand. One hand remains on the controlling rope and is allowed to slide up and down the rope by slackening – but not releasing – grip, while the other hand is used for pulling the rope to the leader through the belay device. A simple procedure is to slide the controlling hand down the rope as far as possible while the other hand grips the rope just above the belay device; the controlling hand then pushes the rope through the device while the other hand pulls it through. A top tip is to keep the belay device pointing upwards in the direction of the leader to prevent snagging.

Most leaders prefer the rope between them and the belayer to have a little slack. A small loop of rope in front of the belayer is adequate: this gives the leader a little room for manoeuvre and offers a good level of security without there being too much slack.

The belayer should stand close to the start of the climb and in a stable and braced position. Standing too far out from the beginning of the climb or way off to the side may well afford a better view of the leader, but introduces dangerous elements into the belay situation by creating the potential for a far longer leader fall than necessary. The shock loading may be enough to drag the belayer towards the bottom of the climb, thus introducing more slack rope into the system plus the possibility that the belayer will lose balance and stumble.

We've already discussed the situations that may require a belayer on the ground to be tied to an upward-pulling anchor when bottom-roping. The merits of employing a similar tactic when belaying a leader are more significant due to the extra forces involved in holding a falling leader compared with a falling second climber.

The key issues to focus on when belaying a leader are as follows:

- **Anticipate the leader's needs** As a good belayer you'll be prepared to pay out the rope or take it in as and when required. For example, if a leader is attempting to clip protection above his head, he'll need a fair bit of rope to do that so the belayer must second guess how much might be needed and pay out the correct amount at just the right moment. The worst-case scenario for a leader is to pull up rope to clip a runner and to find that the belayer hasn't paid out sufficient rope; the rope will suddenly become tight and may be torn from the leader's grasp. This introduces slack rope into the system and if the leader falls at that moment, the chances are that he may fall far enough to suffer a ground fall. When a leader clips into a runner high above his head, at full stretch, the rope will need to be taken in by the belayer in order to prevent a huge amount of slack developing.

- **Organise the rope** Make sure that there are no knots or tangles that might prevent you paying out the rope at a critical moment. There's nothing worse for a leader than to hear words such as 'just hang on a minute while I sort out this mess', because he will know that the belayer's attention will be focussed elsewhere while that's going on.

- **Observe the leader's body language** Being attentive in this way while you're belaying will give you some idea of how the leader is feeling about the climb. If it's very easy, the leader will romp up the climb with confidence. If, however, the leader is finding it difficult, he may make tentative upward moves but then come back down again. And if the leader is scared he may well start shaking – 'sewing machine' leg is a sure sign of a worried leader, as is hugging the rock and displaying a certain amount of reluctance to let go of a substantial handhold. Wise words of encouragement from the belayer are as important in these situations as attention to belaying detail.

- **Communicate well** Be sure to communicate verbally as well as through implicit understanding.

- **Be prepared to hold a fall** It's rare for a leader to fall unexpectedly. Though a foot may suddenly slip or a handhold may snap, when a leader takes a fall there's usually enough build-up to the event to allow the belayer to be well prepared. The action of locking off the belay device to hold a fall must become an ingrained 'automatic reaction' so that if something unexpected happens the belayer has every chance of arresting the fall.

In some situations when a leader falls, it's preferable to apply 'dynamic belay' to arrest the fall. With dynamic belay a small element of extra shock absorption is introduced into holding a fall. When a belay device is locked off to hold a fall, very little rope slippage occurs and the only elements of dynamic belay are the elasticity of the rope and the bodies of the belayer and the leader. While this is significant, it's sometimes desirable to introduce more dynamic belay.

There are two ways to achieve this. One is to allow some rope to 'slip' through the belay device deliberately, but this is incredibly difficult to do; even if you have considerable experience of belaying a leader, things can go horribly wrong if too much rope is allowed to slip. A much better and more controllable method is to lock off the belay device but allow yourself to be pulled slightly towards the base of the climb rather than simply brace against the fall; this takes practice and an indoor venue is much more suitable for this sort of training.

Having mastered belaying a leader indoors, you should move on to outdoor venues. Sport climbs are the easiest style of outdoor climb for this purpose because, compared with trad climbs, they're considerably easier for a leader to protect and security of protection is more predictable.

The detail of leading is considered in the next chapter.

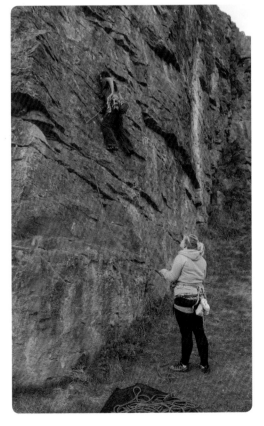

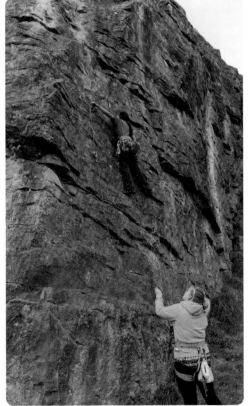

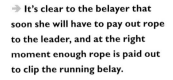
→ **It's clear to the belayer that soon she will have to pay out rope to the leader, and at the right moment enough rope is paid out to clip the running belay.**

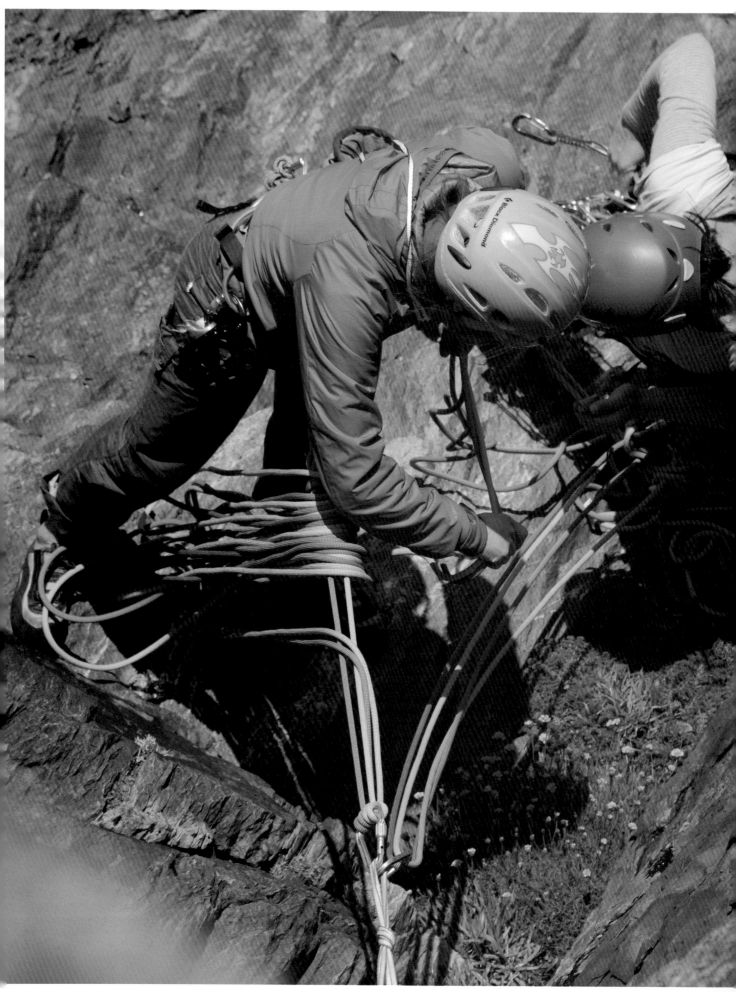

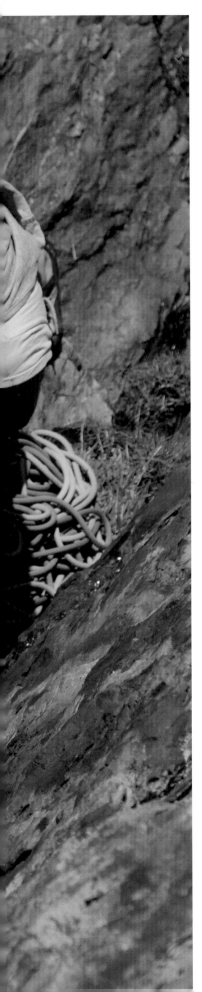

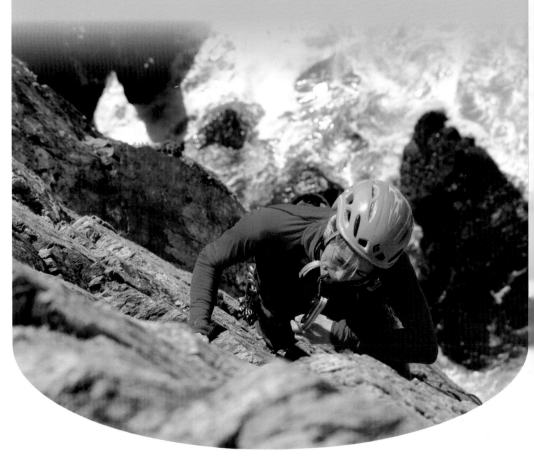

LEADING A CLIMB

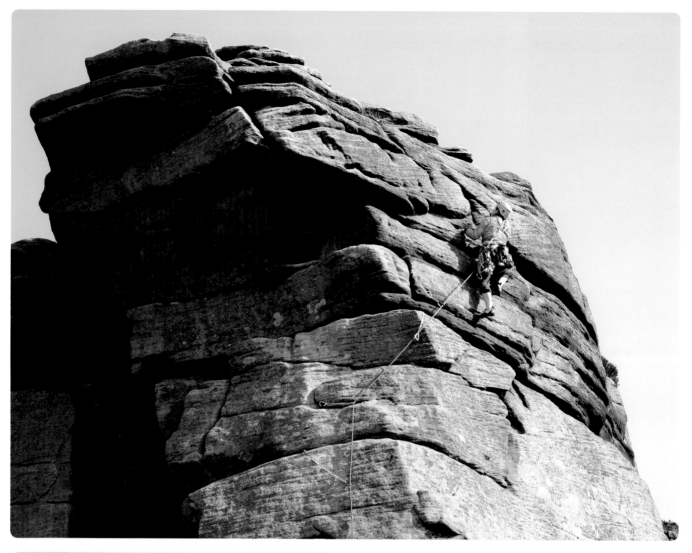

↑ By judicious use of carefully placed running belays the lead climber can arrange protection. Leading a climb carries greater responsibility and risk than climbing with a rope from above so make sure you choose something well within your ability and experience to begin with.

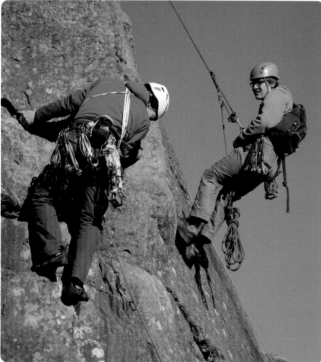

← A climbing instructor ascends a fixed rope alongside a student learning to lead. Remaining in close proximity the instructor is able to offer advice on gear placement and assistance and security if it's required.

A small proportion of people who take up rock climbing have no desire to lead climbs. For others, though, it's the pinnacle of climbing achievement, and pushing the limits of what one can achieve in terms of difficulty and seriousness may be what drives them on.

Fortunately, climbing is a wonderfully fulfilling sport in that the sense of achievement in successfully ascending a climb in good style is attainable whatever grade of difficulty you climb at, from the simplest climb to the most horrendously difficult.

As a leader, being 'the sharp end' of the rope requires a slightly different mindset and approach to simple climbs on a top or bottom rope.

First and foremost, the climber must realise that there's more risk in leading than there is in seconding a climb, where the rope is always above you. Though the risk can be minimised, it cannot be removed entirely. This is what makes rock climbing attractive to some climbers.

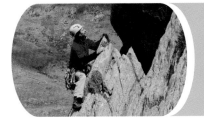

THE LEADING PROCESS

➔ **The Leader of each climbing team will have placed running belays at safe intervals and these are removed by the second as he or she ascends. On longer climbs (multi pitch) the leader is responsible for arranging anchors at each stopping place (stance). Sometimes stances can be very cosy affairs.**

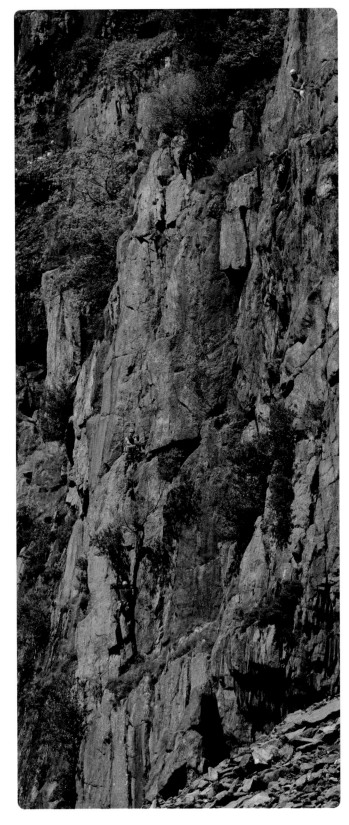

When climbers arrive at a crag, whether a single-pitch sport route or a multi-pitch trad route, someone has to get the rope up the crag in the first instance. This person is the leader.

The leader ascends the chosen route and will either create a sound anchor and bring up the second climber or, on a single-pitch sport route, thread the rope through a fixed 'in-situ' anchor and be lowered back to the ground.

In order to get the rope up in the first place, the climber leads the climbing pitch. If the leader were simply to climb with the rope attached to the harness, placing no protection during the ascent, a fall would almost certainly result in a fall to the ground. In order to prevent this, the leader will place 'running belays' at random intervals – as often as they can be arranged or as often as the leader feels necessary for comfort and safety.

These running belays, which are normally items of crack protection (trad) or bolts (sport) drilled and permanently fixed in the rock, should hold a fall that can be arrested by the belayer, who is known as 'the second'.

In theory, if a leader is 1m above a piece of protection he should only fall 2m (1m to the level of the runner and then 1m below). The reality is that the length of fall will be slightly longer due to the shock absorption properties of the safety system – stretch in the rope,

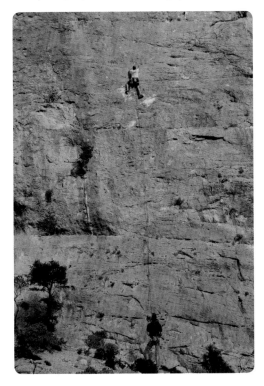

← **Leading a sport climb often feels more comfortable than leading a trad climb because protection is already in place. Though multi-pitch sport routes exist, at a beginner level you're more likely to climb single-pitch routes where you lower back to the ground from the top of the climb.**

tightening of knots and, to a small extent, the dynamic properties of the chosen belaying system.

A leader fall on a trad or sport climb of relatively easy grade is an unusual occurrence. However, circumstances beyond any climber's control may result in a leader fall, so one has to prepare for it as a 'just-in-case' scenario. On considerably more difficult climbs, and particularly where a lead climber is trying something rather harder than he has previously attempted, leader falls will occur more frequently.

Once a climber reaches the heady heights of the higher grades of sport climbs, falling off while leading becomes a given. However, on trad climbs the safety element of a leader fall is entirely dependent on the quality of placement of the protection arranged while on the lead. Tiny micro-wires in a thin, shallow crack are less likely to be able to hold a significant fall than a larger nut or camming device placed in a perfectly tapering crack in sound rock.

The consequences of falling are also dependent on the angle of the rock face being attempted: falling on a low-angled slab of rough rock is more likely to result in injury than a fall on overhanging rock where the climber will hang in space.

Learning to lead climbs safely requires a long apprenticeship and should really be undertaken under expert guidance or at a slow and steady pace where the level of difficulty can increase with experience gained. This chapter should provide a solid grasp of the essentials of leading a climb, but there will be many more scenarios to deal with when leading for real, especially at an advanced level.

Leader falls are best not contemplated on easier climbs that are complicated by ledges and other obstacles, plus the low angle of the rock face.

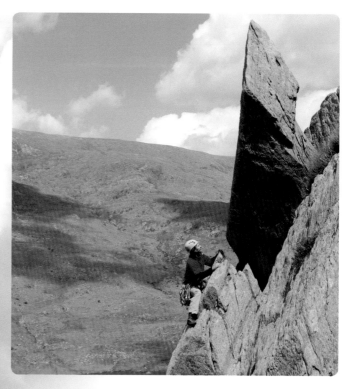

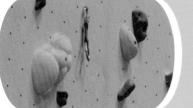

LEADING AT AN INDOOR WALL

An indoor wall is by far the safest place to learn to lead. Protection for the leader is evenly spaced and is arranged so that a ground fall is almost impossible. The quickdraws used for clipping the rope into are nearly always in place and easily clipped on the climb that you're attempting.

The procedure of leading is simple once you've decided on a climb to tackle. The leader ties on to the end of the rope and the belayer places the rope through the belay device. Each then checks that this has been done correctly, that each harness is secured according to the manufacturer's specification, and that the rope is tied into with an appropriate knot. Having done that, you can begin climbing.

As soon as you reach the first quickdraw, clip the rope into it. The second clip is the most critical as it's likely that if you fall while trying to make the second clip you may land on the ground due to the amount of rope out. Once the second clip is made, safety is normally assured!

If possible, try to make each clip when your chest is level with the quickdraw. Making long reaches to attain a clip will provide good protection above your head for much of the climb, but sometimes making long-reach clips into running belays can be quite difficult and tenuous.

The leading progression is as much a learning process for the belayer as it is for the leader. For a novice leader, it may be better to have an experienced belayer on hand to take care of the rope. The belayer must be attentive at all times, watching the leader's every move and trying to anticipate what the leader may need in terms of rope paid out or rope taken in. The ability to predict how much rope a leader will need and when it will be needed is a skill acquired over time and an essential part of the team effort towards climbing safely.

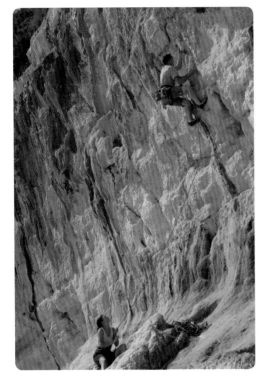

→ **A safe place to learn the basics of leading.**

← **The second clip on any bolt-protected climb is always the most important clip – once done safety is normally assured.**

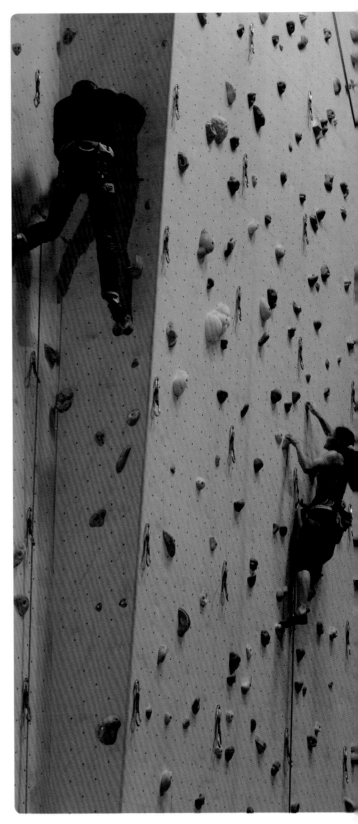

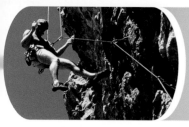
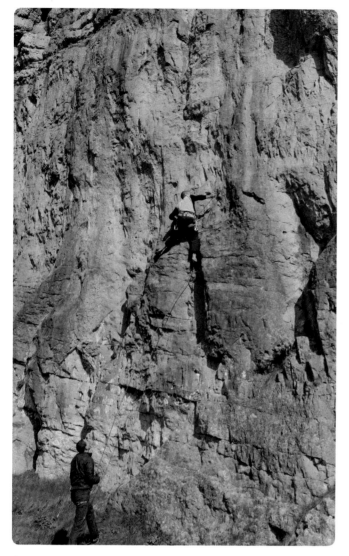

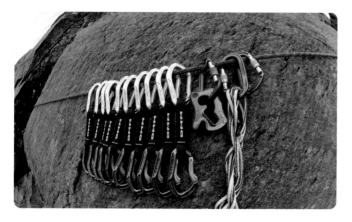

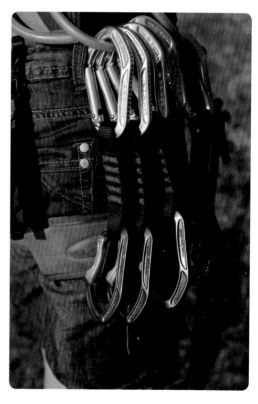

This is broadly the same as leading on an indoor climbing wall, but there are significant differences that make this type of climbing slightly more adventurous.

The main difference is that the quickdraws have to be placed and clipped on the lead. This doesn't sound too troublesome, but sometimes bolt protection is put in places that may not necessarily be comfortable to clip from. You may, for example, have to hang tenuously by your fingertips to make the clip. Quite often the fixed placements aren't as ideally spaced as they might be at an indoor climbing wall.

Three actions are involved: removing the quickdraw from the harness, clipping the quickdraw into the bolt, and then clipping in the rope. Needless to say, it helps to be as efficient as possible.

Quickdraws are carried on the harness gear loops towards the front of the harness so that they're easily accessible. Carrying gear on your harness is termed 'racking'. Spread the quickdraws equally on each side so that if you have, for example, ten draws then put five on each side. Make sure that they're all racked in the same direction, according to personal preference, as this will speed up the whole process and will be much less tiring.

When you clip the quickdraw into the bolt, make sure that both gates of the karabiners face away from the direction that you'll move next. Try to be as slick as you can at clipping in the rope: it's essential to practise this and it can be done while standing firmly on the ground or just a small distance off the ground. There are a number of preferred methods but, like racking, you'll need to discover which suits you best.

⬆ The second clip on this sport climb is quite a long way above the ground and failure to make the clip, though unlikely, might result in a ground fall.

➡ **Quickdraws racked for sport climbing on the harness gear loop. These gates face inwards but some climbers prefer to carry them with gates facing outwards.**

⬅ **A rack of ten quickdraws, a couple of screwgate karabiners, a sling and a belay device (and krab) are all that's required.**

Clipping a quickdraw, first method

1 Pull up the rope, holding it in a loose grip.

2 Put your thumb over the back bar of the karabiner and hold the rope against its gate.

3 The curved gate will allow the rope to slip into the krab, so you don't have to open the gate with your hand.

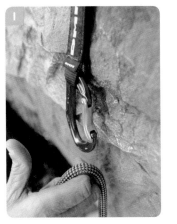
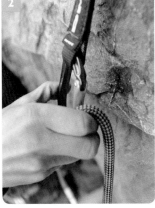
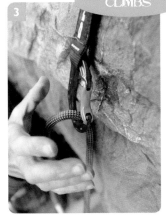

Clipping a quickdraw, second method

1 The second method is similar to the first.

2 But this time the rope is pushed on to the curved karabiner gate…

3 And the rope falls in.

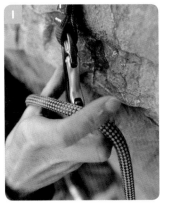
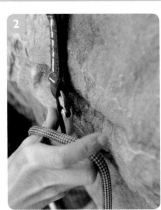
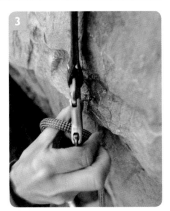

In addition you may find it handy to carry a short sling with a screwgate karabiner for clipping in to the lower-off at the top of the climb while you arrange the rope for the descent. The number of quickdraws you'll carry depends on the length of the pitch and the number of bolts in place. It's always worth carrying a couple more than you actually need for that 'just-in-case' scenario.

If sport climbing is going to be your main sphere of activity, consider buying quickdraws with solid-gate karabiners. These may be fractionally heavier than wire-gate types but are considerably more robust and much less likely to become accidentally twisted when clipped into bolts. Being wider, these quickdraws are also much easier to grab hold of in desperation.

If the climb you're on is only a single pitch and you will lower off from the top, there's no need to carry your belay device.

PLACING PROTECTION

The bolt protection in situ on a sport climb is clipped whenever it's comfortable and desirable to clip! More often than not you'll want to clip from below the bolt and as high up as you can reach. This will mean that you have protection from above for a short section of the climb. However, reaching way above to clip a bolt does have some pitfalls, particularly in situations where you're struggling to hold on.

Clipping a runner high above your head requires a fair amount of rope to be pulled up, usually more than can be pulled up in one arm's length. Thus you have to pull up a bit of rope, hold it in your teeth and then pull up some more so that you can reach the clip. If at the crucial moment your strength fails you and you take a fall, there will be quite a bit of slack rope and the fall will be further than you might expect. Of course, this could have serious implications if the resulting fall means that you hit the ground.

Making a long reach to clip

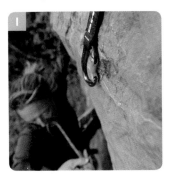
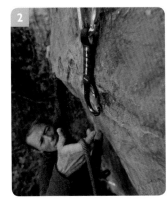
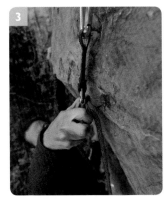
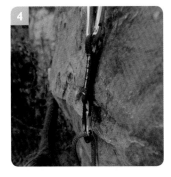

⬆ Pull up a good arm's length of rope and grip it in your teeth.

⬆ Pull up another arm's length of rope.

⬆ Drop the rope from your teeth and reach to make the clip.

⬆ With all clipping methods make sure that the gates of both karabiners face away from the direction you expect to climb.

Using a clip stick

1 A clip stick can be used to make second-bolt clips or even third-bolt clips if you buy a really long one.

2 The quickdraw is retained with the gate open, allowing you to clip it into the bolt.

3 Once the karabiner is in the bolt, hold the climbing rope in one hand (it will be double) and then pull the clip stick away.

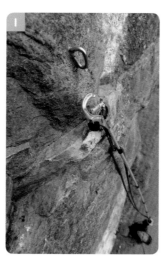

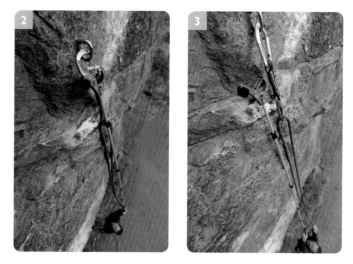

A better tactic is to try to climb a little further before making the clip. As the first couple of clips are the essential ones to make for safety, some climbers use a clip stick to help them clip into the first couple of bolts from the ground. A clip stick is an extendable pole on to which a quickdraw is attached with the gate open and you reach up from the ground to clip in; once the karabiner is in the bolt the clip stick automatically releases.

At the end of the climbing pitch there will be a lower-off point, which can comprise any combination of bolts, chains, fixed karabiners or sometimes rings. Unfortunately there's no set format for lower-offs in the climbing world!

LOWERING OFF

When you've reached the lower-off point at the top of the pitch, the next set of actions will be determined by how your belayer chooses to climb the route, or indeed if he's planning to climb at all.

If your climbing partner is going to do the climb on a rope threaded through the anchor, just attach a quickdraw to each bolt anchor, clip the climbing rope through both and ask your belayer to lower you to the ground. Your partner can then climb the route while you belay from the ground (bottom-roping). It's usually better to leave all quickdraws in place for the second climber to remove during his ascent. On arriving at the lower-off, the second climber can then rig the rope through the fixed anchor and be lowered off. Just to be super-cautious, leave the

final protection bolt on the climb clipped to the rope that goes down to the belayer while you fiddle around setting up the lower-off.

Quite often, one climber will lead a bolted pitch and get lowered off through a couple of quickdraws on the top anchor, leaving all the quickdraws in place. The rope is then pulled through and the second climber can lead the pitch with the benefit of all the quickdraws already in position. On arriving at the top of the climb, the lower-off is rigged so that no gear is left behind, and then the quickdraws are collected on the descent; when both climbers are back on the ground the rope is pulled through and the climb is available for the next team.

Rigging the rope for the lower-off requires great care because eventually the climber will need to untie from the end of the rope. This is the final thing the climber does after checking to see that everything else has been done correctly.

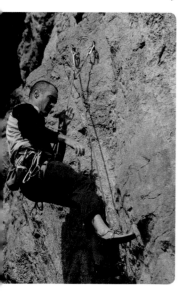

← Two quickdraws through bolts at lower-off.

→ **One climber has already led this sport climb and lowered off from two quickdraws on the lower-off. The next climber has the benefit of the quickdraws already in place. A long sling has been clipped to one of the bolts to provide protection between two otherwise widely spaced bolts.**

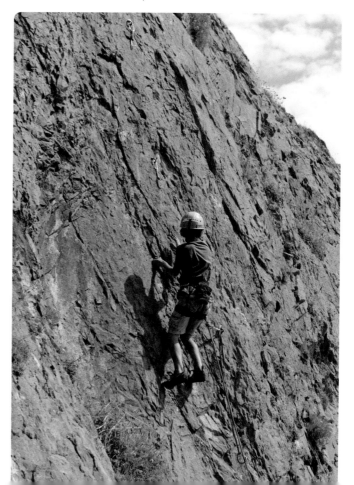

Rigging a lower-off

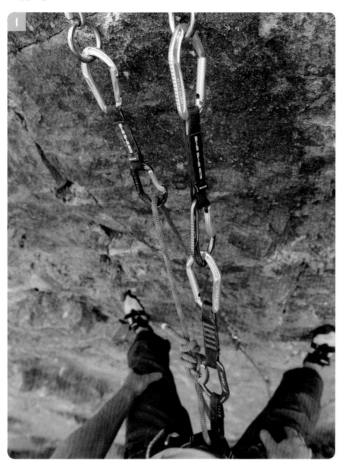

↑ One of the lower-off anchors is used for a runner and the belayer takes in the rope tight while the climber clips into the other anchor with a quickdraw or, as illustrated here, two quickdraws; provided that the climber keeps these under tension it's safe enough. At this point the belayer can relax and slacken off the rope in anticipation of the next step.

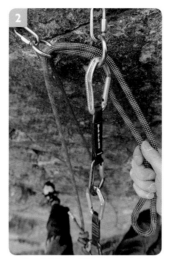

↑ The leader takes a bight of rope and threads it through both rings of the lower-off.

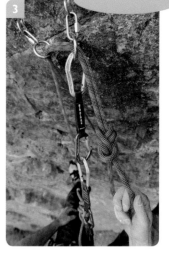

↑ And then ties a figure eight on the bight…

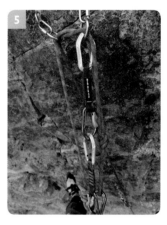

↑ …and clips to the harness belay loop using a screwgate karabiner.

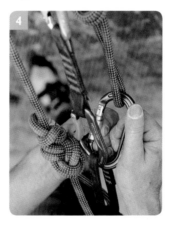

↑ Before untying the end of the rope, check that everything is threaded correctly.

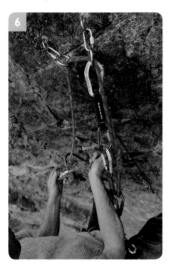

↑ Next, untie from the end of the rope.

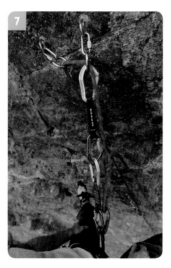

↑ The belayer now takes the weight of the leader once again.

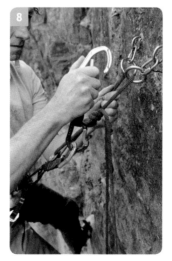

↑ Before unclipping the quick draws check that the belayer is ready to lower and that the lower-off is threaded correctly.

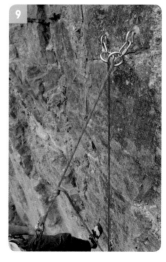

↑ And down you go…

Rigging a lower-off with a cowstail

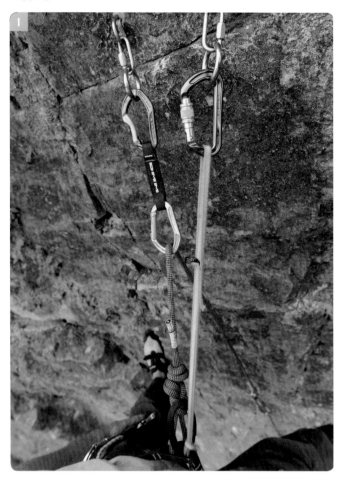

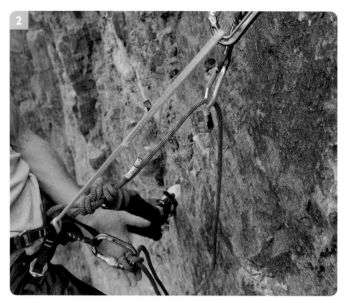

⬆ Take up some slack rope and secure it to the belay loop on the harness with a clove hitch.

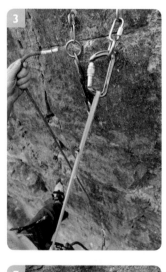

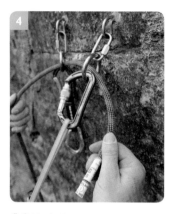

⬆ Some climbers prefer to rig a lower-off with a cowstail. As with the previous method, clip one of the lower-off anchors as a runner and ask the belayer to take your weight. Make up a cowstail using a short sling and then clip into the lower-off with a screwgate karabiner; the belayer can relax a bit at this point.

⬅⬆ Untie from the end of the rope, then thread it through both lower-off rings…

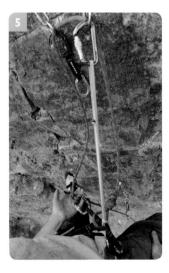

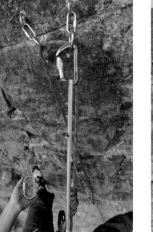

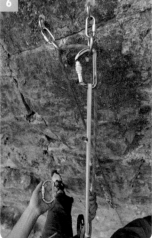

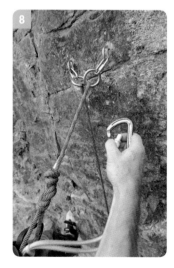

⬆ …and then tie back into the harness as normal.

⬆ Release the clove hitch from the krab on the belay loop.

⬆ Ask the belayer to take your weight and double-check that you've done everything correctly before you unclip the cowstail.

⬆ Unclip the cowstail and down you go…

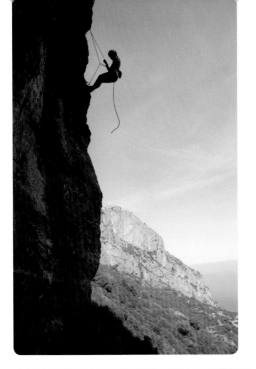

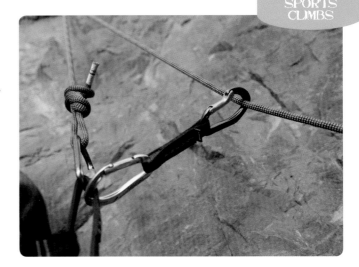

←↓→ **On sport climbs that go diagonally across the face or up overhanging rock, you may need to hold yourself into the rock in order to reach the quickdraws to clear them – this is known as tramming. It can be quite strenuous and you need to consider the implications of unclipping the final quickdraw on the way down.**

It's essential to practise the lowering-off process in a safe place before you need to do it for real. An indoor wall may have the facility to practise such rope techniques.

MAKING A COWSTAIL

A cowstail is a simple method of creating an attachment loop that can be used to clip into anchor points in place of the rope.

There are slings called 'daisychains' that have several sewn loops along their length, offering the facility to vary the length of the cowstail attachment with ease. You can also create a cowstail using a long sling.

The accompanying photos show a cowstail attachment threaded through the harness tie-in loops and larksfooted back on itself. A knot has been tied a few centimetres from the end and this could be used if a shorter attachment is necessary. It's also easy to move the knot along for an even shorter attachment. A suggested method of storing the cowstail when it isn't being used, but when you anticipate needing it again a little later, is also illustrated.

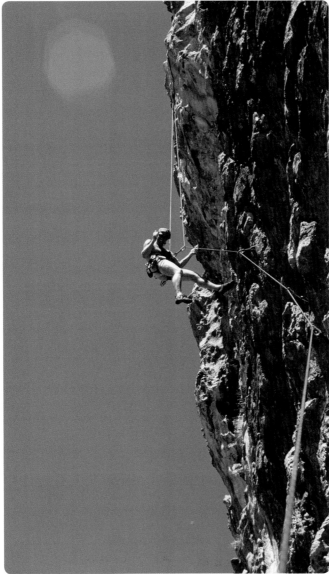

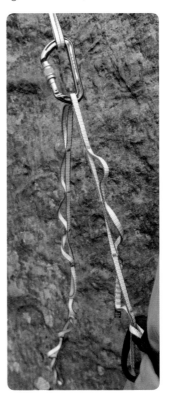

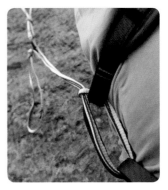

⬆ **Cowstail sling.**

⬅ **Cowstail daisychain.**

⬇ **Cowstail stowed.**

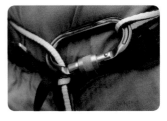

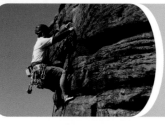

LEADING TRAD CLIMBS

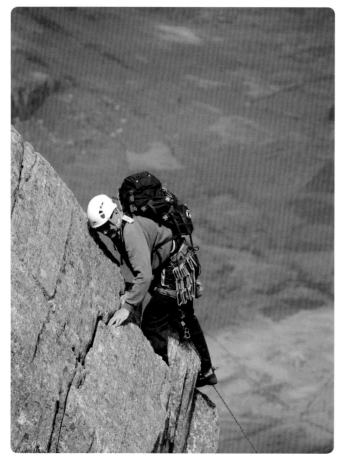

↑ 'Real' Trad climbing high on a mountain face. A long approach walk and the need to carry everything with you on the climb make it a big mountain day out.

↓ A suitable selection of gear for the novice leader, but there are many options. Some experienced climbers would say that camming devices and very tiny nuts on wire are unnecessary at beginner level. What you select in the end will also be driven by budget.

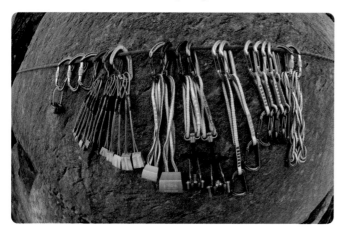

This is considerably more involved than any other of the previously described styles of leading climbs, the most significant difference being the amount of kit you'll require.

Learning to use all the equipment and the responsibilities of leading is best achieved in a safe environment with professional instruction, where the instructor is attached to a separate rope and ascends alongside the student climber. The instructor will normally climb the pitch first, attach a rope to an anchor at the top of the pitch, abseil down to the student climber, and then ascend the fixed rope alongside the student, using mechanical devices. Should assistance be required, the instructor can offer it at any time.

Most, but not all, trad climbs are more than one pitch in length. Any climb that ascends in two or more stages is called multi-pitch. There are various factors that determine the length of a pitch:

■ Convenience of stopping places with suitable anchors.
■ Changes of direction in the route to be taken.
■ The length of the climbing rope.

Pitches, therefore, could be as short as a few metres or the full length of the rope available. At the end of each pitch the leader will arrange an anchor and bring up the second climber to the stance. Before you actually embark on the climb you'll decide whether the same person will lead all of the pitches or you will swap leads and share the responsibility. The first tactic is usually used for climbing partnerships where one of the team doesn't want to lead or isn't experienced enough to lead. The second tactic, known as sharing the lead or leading through, is applicable to teams of more or less equal ability where both would like to lead, and is more efficient for longer climbs.

All of the safety equipment that you'll use on a climb will be placed by the leader during ascent and removed by the second climber. We've already discussed the different types of crack protection and sling placement when creating anchors (see Chapter 5) and exactly the same principles apply to placing gear on the lead. There are, however, external factors that may make it slightly trickier to arrange protection than on a practice boulder or small crag; the most notable difference is that you may find yourself hanging on with one hand and needing to place protection with the other. This is why it's far better to learn on low-angle, easy climbs where you're more likely to be able to take two hands off the rock to deal with gear placements.

GEAR REQUIRED

Much less kit is needed for easy climbs than for climbs higher up the grades. All the crack protection, slings, karabiners and quickdraws you'll need are collectively referred to as the 'rack'.

A suitable rack for climbs of lower grades (say up to V Diff) will normally be made up of a selection of nuts (wedges and hexes) from sizes 1 through to 9 or 10. Camming devices aren't essential, though it's likely that most climbers starting out will want to have a couple on their rack. If you're such a climber, consider getting sizes 2 and 3 as these will probably be the most useful, and you can add to them as you gain experience and begin to climb harder routes.

➡ **There are several ways to rack gear on your harness gear loops. Here wires of similar size are grouped in bunches on the climber's right side. Karabiners holding all the gear are racked facing inwards or outwards according to personal preference.**

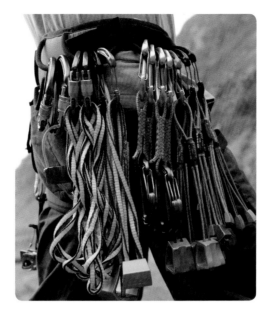

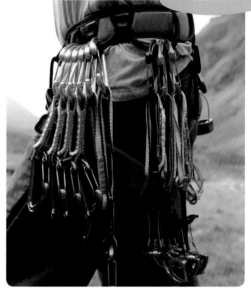

➡➡ **A selection of cams racked on the same climber's left side. Notice how in both photos there's order to the racking, to this climber's preference: wires are racked small to big towards the back, and cams small to big.**

RACKING

The most common method of carrying gear is by racking, with all crack protection, quickdraws, spare karabiners and your belay device carried directly on the gear loops of the harness. The right harness for trad climbing has a reasonably substantial waist belt combined with a good selection of gear loops on the sides and at the back. A harness designed specifically for sport climbing is usually too lightweight and flimsy to carry the heavier rack of gear needed for trad climbing, and this extra weight may drag such a harness down over the hips; in addition sport-climbing harnesses won't have many gear loops.

Having selected a rack, the next decision is how to carry it. Nuts are normally carried on a single karabiner and grouped in similar sizes. It's a good idea not to have too many nuts on a krab, say four or five at most. If you group nuts in similar sizes, when you come to place one in a crack you may not get the correct size immediately but at least you'll have a choice of similar sizes already in your hand – this kind of efficient organisation of your equipment will save you considerable energy in the long run. When a nut is placed in a crack it can be firmly seated by a

sharp tug on the remaining bunch of nuts. The next step is to take the bunch off the placed nut, return them to the gear loop and then take a quickdraw to clip the rope into the placement. You'll need to clip a quickdraw into the wire runner in order to reduce leverage on the wire caused by the friction of the rope running through a karabiner.

To further improve the efficiency of gear placements, there are other considerations. Just as with racking quickdraws for sport climbing, rack all karabiners with the gate facing the same way, inwards or outwards according to your preference. If you also rack your kit in exactly the same order and the same place on your harness every time, you'll come to know precisely where to reach for any particular item. This will make an enormous difference to the efficiency with which you climb, particularly in stressful situations.

Though it's used much less frequently nowadays, another method is to carry some of your kit on a bandolier, which is something of an acquired taste but has several advantages. Perhaps the most significant advantage is that you won't have such a heavy weight hanging from your harness. Climbers who use bandoliers normally carry all their

➡ **Having placed a nut in the crack, this climber returns his bunch of nuts to the harness, in the correct place.**

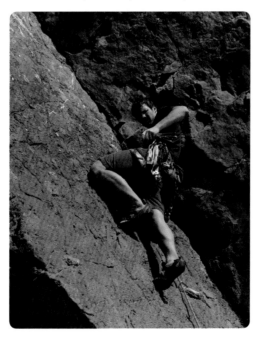

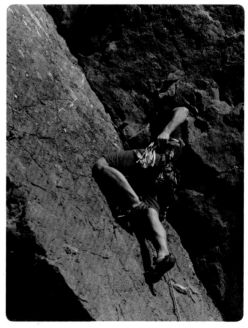

➡➡ **A quickdraw is taken from the harness, clipped to the wire and then the rope is clipped in. Wire-slung nuts need to be extended with a quickdraw to reduce leverage that might otherwise lift the nut out of the crack. For trad climbing, wire-gate snaplink krabs are ideal.**

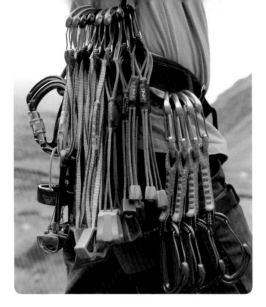

← Some climbers like to have gear racked on a bandolier, a method that's particularly useful when you have to carry a lot of kit.

crack protection gear – the bulk of the weight of the total rack – attached to the bandolier, and the suggested method is shown in the accompanying photo. Another advantage of using a bandolier is for swapping over gear on stances when you lead through with your partner; the bandolier can be exchanged between the climbers and the rack rearranged as necessary.

As a beginner, it will take time to develop your preferences in

racking, but it's important to do your experimentation with various systems before settling for what works well for you. Many people regard a bandolier as 'old school', but if, as a beginner, you have the opportunity to experiment with one you may find that you grow to like the system.

PLACING PROTECTION

The frequency of runner placements on trad climbs will be determined largely by their availability. A climb that follows a crack system in the rock is likely to have plenty of such opportunities, whereas a climb that ascends a blank-looking slab may have few crack features.

Assuming that you could pick and choose when to place protection on the lead, you would ideally place it as often as possible all the way up the pitch. If you find a climb particularly easy there may be a temptation to place less protection, which is all very heroic but takes no account of the consequences of an accidental slip or misjudgement – so to fully respect team safety at least some protection should always be placed.

The best place to practise placing protection is while you're comfortably standing on terra firma. Find a piece of rock or a boulder that has a variety of cracks and fissures and experiment at will with types of placement. Taking this further, you can step up off the ground and hang on with one hand while placing gear, trying this with a selection of gear on your harness, as if in a 'real' climbing situation. Practice like this will pay dividends in the end. The detail of placement is covered in Chapter 5.

← Plenty of protection here – six running belays within four or five metres.

⬇ The importance of placing a running belay as soon as possible after leaving a stance cannot be stressed too highly. In this photo, taken on a multi-pitch sport climb, one of the anchor bolts has been used as a runner to prevent a leader fall directly on to the belayer.

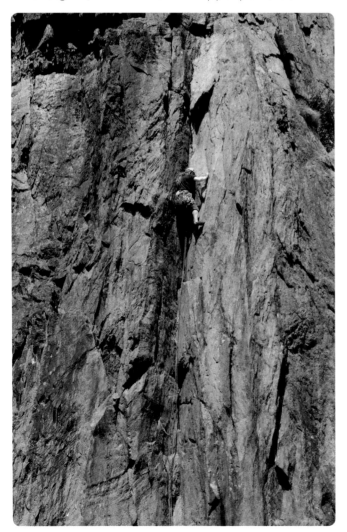

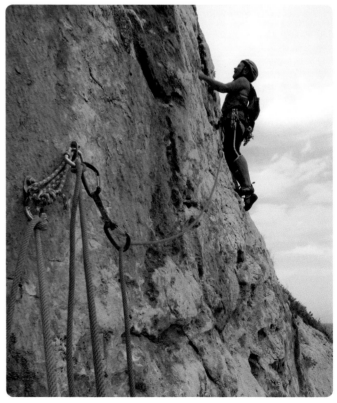

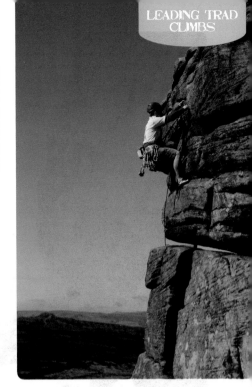

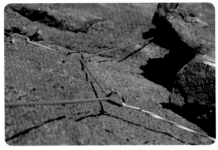

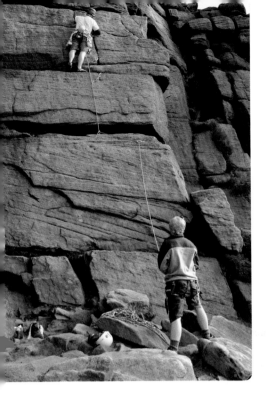

⬆ **Runners extended, one with a long quickdraw, the other with a long sling. Even so, there's still a bit of drag created by the bends in the rope.**

⬅ **This climber will almost certainly find it difficult to pull the rope through the runners. The only solution to this problem is to use double ropes or leave out the right-hand runner.**

➡ **The nut placement in the horizontal crack has been extended so that no drag is created.**

The reality of gear placement for leader protection is that whenever a good placement presents itself you should consider putting something in. There are a few occasions when it's vital to place gear whether you feel the need for it or not. Two such scenarios are as follows:

■ At the beginning of a climb where the terrain below the crag is steep.
■ As soon as possible after leaving the stance on multi-pitch climbs.

This safety procedure prevents the possibility of a leader falling with the force fully taken by the belayer. For example, consider the situation on the second pitch of a climb where the leader is 4m above the belayer on the stance. The leader will fall a total of 8m and this fall will have to be held directly by the belayer on to his harness and anchor attachment. This is known as a fall factor of 2: the calculation is made by dividing the distance of the fall (8m) by the amount of rope paid out (4m). The amount of stress that a fall factor of 2 generates is the maximum strain that can be placed on the climbing safety chain and as such it's perfectly possible that some part of the chain could fail.

Take the same scenario but with a sound running belay placed 3m above the belayer. Here the leader fall will only be 2m, giving a fall factor of 0.5

Using the formula, you can see that it's possible to take quite large falls if there's more rope between each climber. For example, if a leader is 30m above the belayer with a runner at 25m, the fall will be 10m; this is a very long fall but the fall factor in this case is only 0.3.

In an ideal world running belay protection should be placed every two or three metres. Occasionally you may feel the need for more, particularly when faced with the most difficult section of a climb, called the crux. Prior to making the difficult move, the leader may place two or three pieces of protection in close proximity to each other. This gives a morale boost and makes the moves seem so much easier. Protection can be a great comfort.

Inevitably there'll be times when it's tricky to get protection where and when you'd like it. That's the spicy bit about climbing. Marginal or dodgy placements abound and very occasionally the leader will place something that's merely psychological. If it's enough to help you overcome a section of particularly challenging climbing without falling off, then it will have served a useful purpose.

You will need to consider the implications of placing protection on pitches that meander their way up a section of rock or where running belays can only be found to one side or another of the route up. When you climb with a single rope it's possible that clipping runners off each side will result in the rope running up the cliff in a zigzag line, which has two rather undesirable effects, as follows:

■ It will introduce rope drag, which in an extreme case can be so severe that upward movement becomes nigh on impossible. Not only might you have to pull yourself up the rock, but you'll also be pulling against the friction created by the rope.
■ When you inadvertently create rope drag, protection you have placed on the ascent could be pulled out. Obviously this is a rather uncompromising position to be in, particularly if the gear that comes out is crucial to safety.

Try to arrange protection so that the climbing rope runs as straight as possible between leader and belayer. Often this can be achieved simply enough by extending running belays using quickdraws of varying lengths.

To help alleviate the problem of rope drag climbers use double ropes, a procedure that's discussed in detail later in this chapter. The basic premise is that one rope is clipped to runners on the left and the other to runners on the right.

There are occasions when it's sensible to place running belays in consideration of the second climber. An example of this scenario is where a pitch goes fairly straight for much of its length but the final part on to the belay ledge or stance necessitates a traverse to the left or right. A traverse of only 1–2m doesn't present too much of a problem, but one that's 5–6m is altogether different.

Traverses can be quite intimidating for the second climber, so prudent placement of running belays will be much appreciated. Try to get a running belay at the very beginning of the traverse and maybe one or two more along the traverse line. Though this will probably introduce some rope drag, the safety it provides usually outweighs that slight disadvantage.

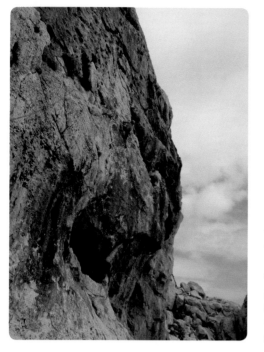

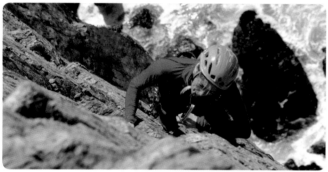

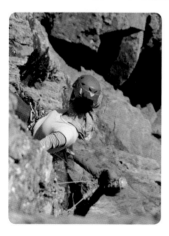

← The second climber always appreciates protection on a traverse. Here it would have been very easy for the leader to neglect to place a runner at the start of the short traverse, in which case the second climber might face the prospect of a swing were he or she to fall at that point.

⬆ If you're hanging on with one hand and trying to arrange protection with the other, you can hold gear in your teeth!

← Communication between leader and second is vital. Sometimes neither will be able to see the other and it may be difficult to work out what's going on. At times like these the second needs patience and understanding.

Placing running belays on the lead can sometimes be awkward. You may find yourself in an uncomfortable and strenuous position, holding on with the fingertips of one hand and reluctant to let go of the rock with the other in order to arrange protection. In these situations gripping gear in your teeth can provide a handy tool! This is useful for holding a bunch of wires while you select the correct size, or you can climb down to a more comfortable point to select the gear and then climb back up with the chosen item gripped between your teeth. Just remember not to begin a conversation with your belayer before you've taken the gear out of your mouth!

Teeth are also useful for gripping the rope when you have to make a long reach to clip a runner. You can pull up a short section of rope, grip it between your teeth and then pull up more. If you slip off during this process don't forget to release the rope as you fall…

Communication with your climbing partner is essential throughout the whole process.

LEADING USING DOUBLE-ROPE TECHNIQUE

On more straightforward climbs using a single rope for safety is perfectly adequate. As you progress through the grades, however, it's likely that you'll need to branch out into using two ropes.

There are distinct advantages to double-rope technique and only one minor disadvantage – it requires a little more care in managing ropes. Some of the key advantages are as follows:

■ It's easier to arrange protection to either side of the actual route.
■ If a pitch of the climb meanders around, there's less likelihood of creating rope drag.
■ If alternate runners are clipped into each of the ropes, there'll always be a protective runner to hold you if you fall while clipping the next.
■ You can descend further by abseil when using double ropes (see Chapter 8).

Climbers who use double-rope technique will usually choose ropes with a diameter of 9mm or slightly less, and I think rope of around 8.5mm diameter is ideal. It's a good idea to have different colours of rope so that they can be easily identified. The UIAA designation for a suitable rope for double-rope technique is ½ rope, but don't confuse this with the requirements of twin-rope technique, where two very thin 7mm ropes are used but are treated as a single rope in terms of climbing safety techniques. It isn't always an advantage to climb with the thinnest ropes available in the ½ rope category as they can sometimes be a little too thin for good grip. Only go for the thinner

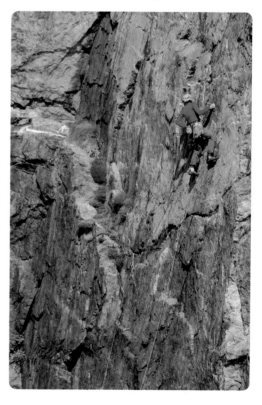

→ The use of double ropes allows the leader to place protection on a climb that meanders around. A good deal of thought needs to go into the best way to utilise each rope and no two pitches will ever be the same.

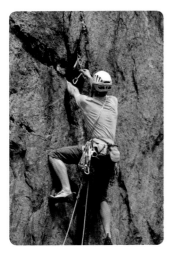

⬆ **One advantage of double ropes is safety. It's possible to place a runner and clip into it while still benefiting from the security of the second rope through a runner.**

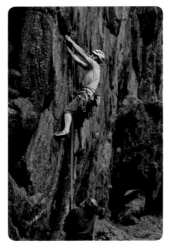

⬆ **The safety advantage of double ropes is nowhere better illustrated than low down on the climb where moves may be quite difficult. An attentive, alert and competent second is vital.**

➡ **Nicely organised at the start of the climb, with ropes sorted out on the ground and totally free of tangles. It's vital to spend time organising equipment as you climb – you'll encounter far fewer problems.**

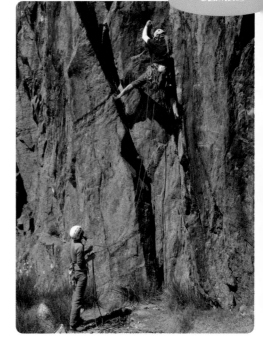

style when weight is important, such as on a big adventure climb in a remote area that necessitates a long walk in.

One simple rule must be observed when using double ropes. Always clip the same rope to runners on the left and the other rope to runners on the right, though in practice this may not prove to be straightforward. It's usually quite difficult to predict before setting out on a pitch exactly where runners will be found and this will often result in placements that are inconsistently left or right of the actual line taken. There's no golden rule to overcome this and mostly you'll just have to work it out as you climb. Occasionally this might mean that you'll have to clip one rope into a sequence of runners, saving the other for when it's needed further up the pitch, where, again, you may have to clip into a sequence of placements.

It's very easy to get the ropes twisted around each other. The simplest and most innocuous way that this happens is on a stance where you may, without necessarily being aware of it, step over something and turn round. This doesn't matter if you then reverse the movement, but if you do a similar thing a second time you'll instantly have two twists in your two ropes.

It's much more important to run the ropes through on each stance if you're not leading through, and, if possible, run each of the ropes through individually. Obviously if you're leading through this action isn't usually required.

KEEPING ROPES FREE OF TANGLES
This is an often-overlooked but essential practice. It takes time but if you sort out ropes carefully it will prevent a problem arising at an inopportune moment.

When the leader is belaying the second climber up the pitch, all the rope taken in will lie in a pile on the ledge. The second climber will reach the stance and secure himself to the anchor. If the second climber isn't going to lead the next pitch, the end of the rope to which the leader is attached will be at the bottom of the pile. The second climber, therefore, should run the rope through, reversing the pile so that the leader's end of the rope is on top and the rope will run smoothly out for the following pitch.

Problems of rope organisation are compounded if there is no suitable ledge for the rope to be piled upon. It's not a good idea to allow the rope simply to drape down the cliff face. A loop of rope may snag itself on a protrusion, especially if blown around by a strong breeze.

In these situations, most often encountered on small and narrow ledges or on hanging stances, it's good practice to lap the rope over your tie-in to the anchor. The length of the laps can vary according to the situation but the golden rule is that they mustn't hang down the crag too far below you. Longer laps mean fewer laps over the anchor tie-in and are possibly more manageable than many shorter laps.

⬇ **There's no ledge here to provide time and room to sort yourself out, and an incoming tide increases the pressure to hasten along. So each of the two climbing ropes is lapped around the feet, which is a great idea but doesn't allow much wriggle room if you get cramp through remaining in the same position for a long time.**

⬊ **A hanging stance is one where there's no ledge to stand on and sometimes not even a foothold. If the ropes will hang into open air you can make the lapped coils fairly long.**

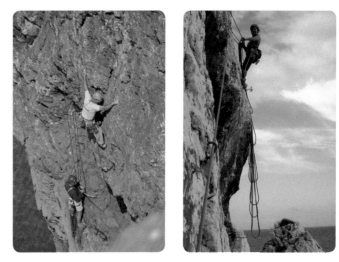

THE SECOND CLIMBER'S ROLE

Though this chapter is about leading a climb, the whole process is a team effort both in terms of safety and efficient movement. As such the second climber – known as the 'second' – has an important role to play, so a few top tips won't go amiss.

The second has the responsibility of removing all gear from the climb so that nothing gets left behind as the climbing team progresses up the route. Sounds simple enough!

All the gear that's removed needs to be stored on the harness. When a runner with a quickdraw attached is removed, clip the middle karabiner to the gear loop on your harness or bandolier. If you clip the end krab, it will dangle down well below your knees and just get in the way. Slings are most efficiently carried around the shoulder.

Removing protection isn't always straightforward. The tactic is to take a quick look at how it might have gone in and, once you have an idea of that, try to loosen the nut with your fingers and then simply lift it out of the crack, with a sharp tap from the end of the nut key if necessary. If that doesn't release the protection, you may have to use a little more force.

← **Trying to remove gear placed by the leader can be extremely tiring and frustrating for a second. If the protection is wedged tightly in the crack, two hands may be required to loosen and remove it, and this can only be done by the belayer taking the weight of the second on the rope.**

⬇ **When removing a camming device from a placement, make sure that you fully close the cams so that the device can be removed easily. If the runner has been extended, as seen here, take the cam off the extender, clip it to your harness and arrange the sling around your shoulder to store it out of the way.**

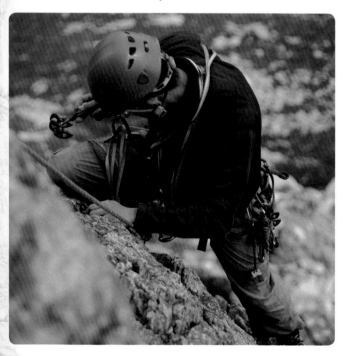

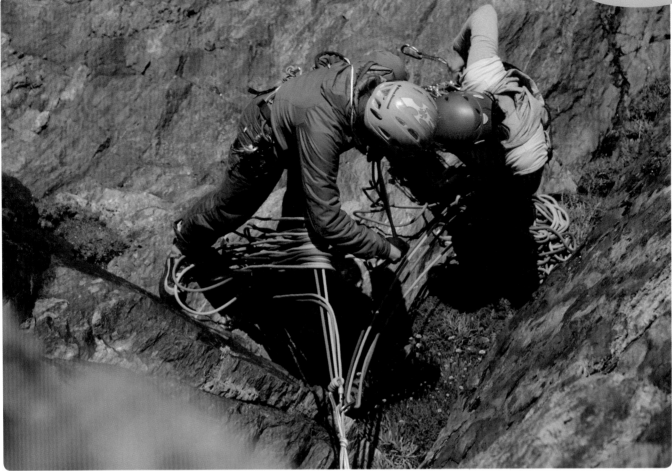

Removing a camming device is usually the reverse of placing it: grab the finger pull, put the thumb on the bar end, squeeze until the cams close, then lift it out. If a camming device becomes completely wedged or has 'walked' deeper into the crack, you may not be able to get your fingers on the trigger bar. The worst-case scenario is one where the cam is buried deep in the crack and the cams have either opened out completely or become totally closed. Two hands will be required in this situation, so ask your leader to take your body weight on the rope. You'll be able to focus all your attention on the extraction rather than worry about hanging on with waning strength.

When the second finally reaches the leader on the stance, the first thing to do is to secure to the anchor. If you're taking over the lead, this need only be a temporary measure so use a cowstail or a clove hitch in the rope anchored with a screwgate karabiner. On the other hand, if you'll be seconding again, the tie-in needs to be more permanent so take time to ensure it's done correctly.

As soon as you're secured begin sorting out the rack of gear. This basically means rearranging it so that it's systematically racked just as at the beginning of the climb. Determining how it's racked depends on who will lead the next pitch, as gear is always racked to the leader's preference. If the stance is small and airy, gear can be exchanged by clipping it on to the rope to the anchor tie-in.

Paying out double ropes can be slightly trickier than a single rope. As with any belaying scenario, you must always keep control of the dead or slack rope. Having two ropes to handle makes this awkward, particularly when you may need to pay out one rope but not the other. The accompanying photo shows a suggested grip on paying the rope out to the leader.

↑ **Organising equipment at a stance: while one climber laps the ropes over the connections to the anchor, the other is sorting out the gear collected on the previous pitch. Efficiencies in the way you manage stances and changeovers will come with experience.**

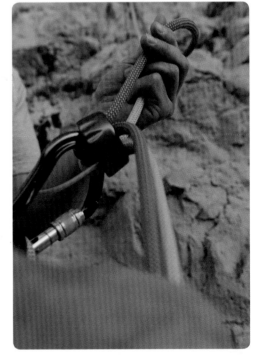

→ **Paying out double rope requires some dexterity. It's really important not to let go of the controlling ropes at any time. The best solution is to try to keep a slackened grip around the control ropes and use the fingers and thumb to pull out either of the ropes as may be needed by the leader.**

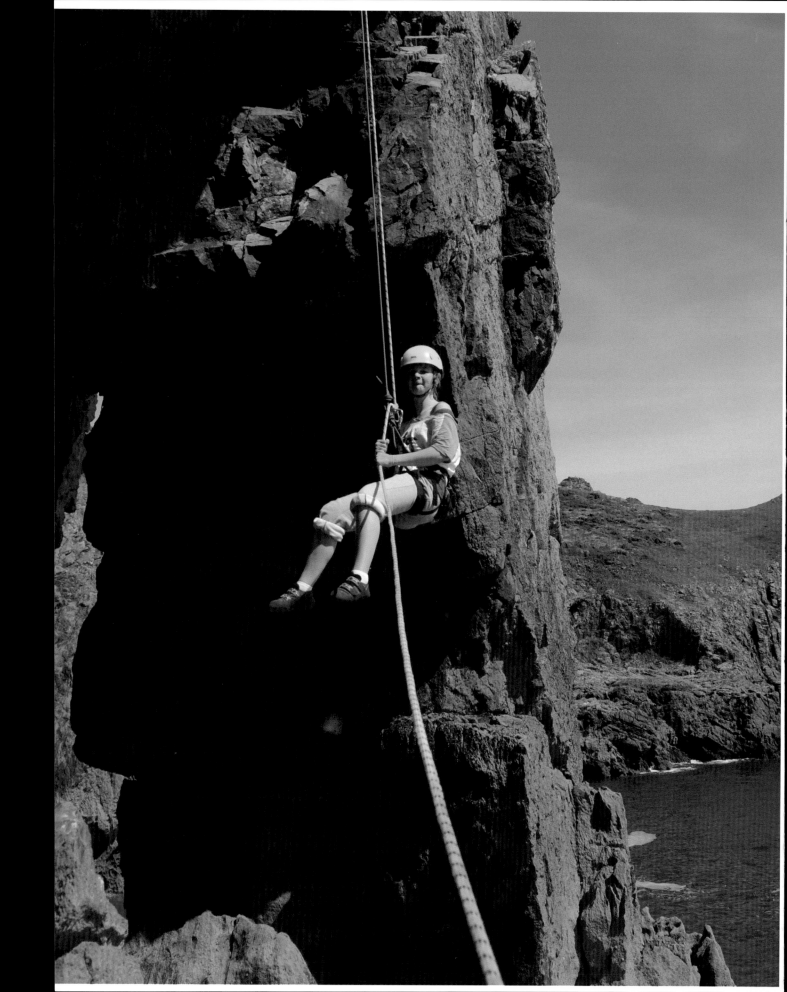

ABSEILING

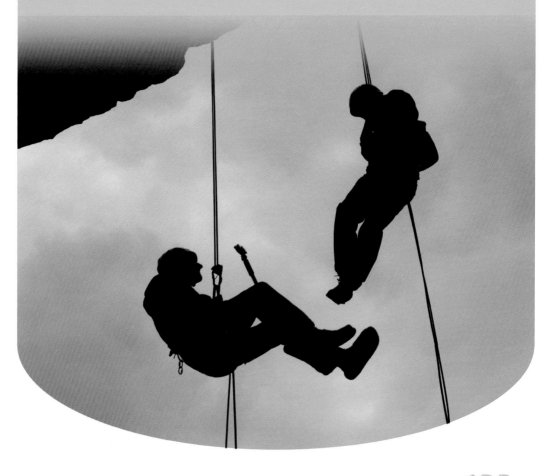

There are many reasons why climbers will need to abseil and it's essential to understand the techniques required and to practise the different methods in a controlled environment before using them in day-to-day climbing.

Abseiling is used as a means of descent from the top of some climbs. There are crags and cliffs where fixed abseil anchors are permanently in place to facilitate this. On many crags a single 50m abseil will get you back on the ground but there are just as many where multiple abseil descents may be required. The possibility also exists where much of the descent may be by walking or scrambling with a short abseil necessary at some point along the way.

If, for whatever reason, you're forced to retreat from a climb it's likely that you'll need to do so by abseil. If the reason for retreat has an element of urgency about it, great care and caution should be exercised.

If you climb on cliffs above the sea it's very likely that an abseil descent from the top of the cliff to the base at sea level will be the only access to the climb. This may present other issues that need dealing with, such as making a belay anchor and sorting gear and ropes so that they don't fall into the water.

Whatever the reason for abseiling, the techniques vary little and attention to detail needs to be an absolute priority regardless of whether the abseil is long or short.

⬅ **Abseil descent from the Old Man of Hoy in the Orkney Islands, Scotland – not a good place for your first practice abseil!** *(© Gary Smith)*

⬇ **There are many reasons why climbers may need to abseil. The two most common are a descent from the top of a climb (to save a long walk in uncomfortable rock shoes) and to access climbs on sea cliffs.**

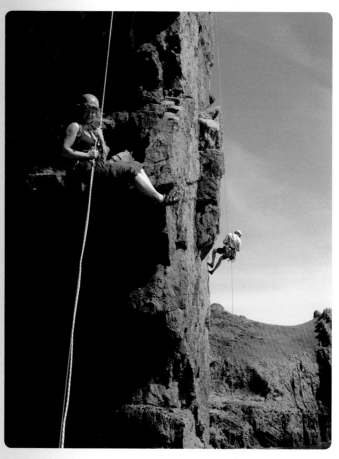

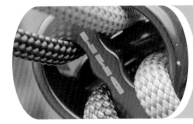

TECHNIQUE AND EQUIPMENT

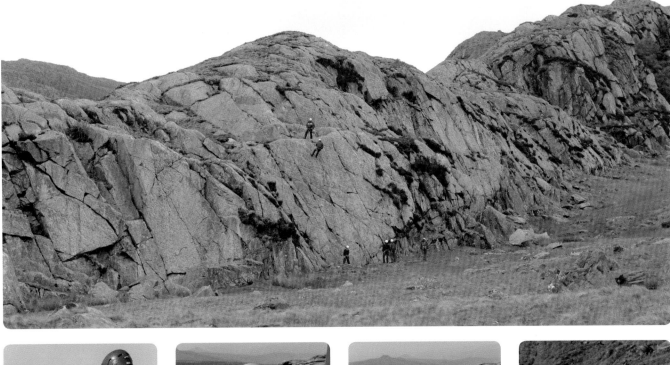

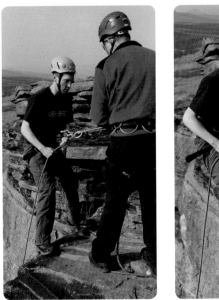 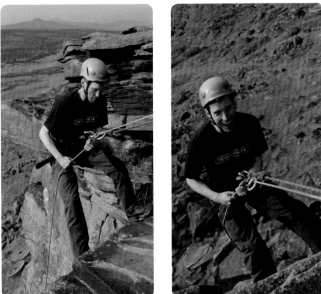

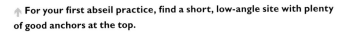
⬆ **For your first abseil practice, find a short, low-angle site with plenty of good anchors at the top.**

If, as a novice climber, you own a belay device, screwgate karabiners and slings, you'll have all the tools needed to abseil. The only extra bit of kit that will be useful is a Prusik loop (see Chapter 4).

To begin learning the techniques required to abseil, you should try to find a low-key venue. A great place to start is a single-pitch crag where you're also able to practise other climbing techniques. You can go to the top of the crag to rig anchor points, link them all together and attach a rope, which can then be hung down the crag.

If possible, make the first few descents with a safety rope attached to your harness. To do this, you'll need to have someone belay the safety rope and this person will in turn need to be secured to the anchors. The safety rope can be secured with a traditional belaying method or by a direct belay using an Italian hitch.

The belay device is excellent for abseiling as it provides more than

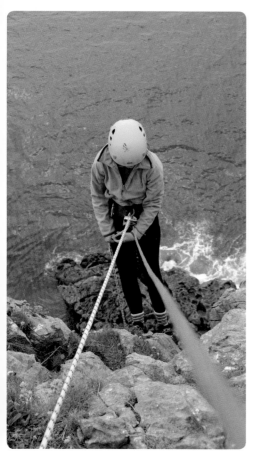

← **Use a safety rope until you gain confidence. Here the safety rope is tied into the harness tie-in points, as for climbing.**

→ **Try to keep the feet flat on the rock and the legs perpendicular to the rock face – this is perfect.**

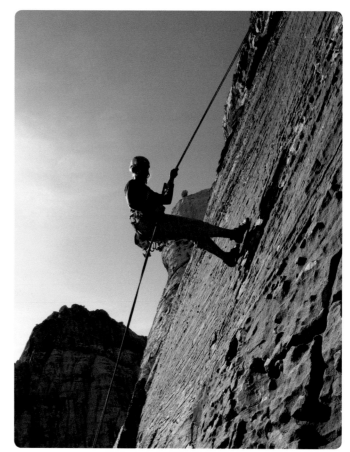

sufficient friction to control the speed of descent. It's attached to the belay/abseil loop of the harness as illustrated. The safety rope can be tied directly into the harness or clipped into the belay/abseil loop using a figure of eight on the bight clipped to a screwgate karabiner.

The technique for descending is simple enough. Keep all your weight on the rope, place your feet flat against the rock face and lean backwards. The most difficult part of abseiling is actually getting started. It helps in a practice session if the rope to the anchor is way above the starting point of the abseil, as this makes it considerably easier to get all your weight on the rope and start moving.

Keeping a firm grip on the controlling rope, you gradually allow the rope to slide through the belay device. As you do so, walk your feet down a bit at a time. The ideal speed at which to descend is determined by the rate at which the rope is allowed to slide through your hands combined with the need for your feet to keep pace. Always try to keep feet flat on the rock and legs perpendicular to the angle of the rock face.

It's important to stress here that abseiling in 'commando' style is considered dangerous in a rock-climbing environment. You don't need to rush down the cliff or face outwards to fire a weapon at the enemy below. In fact, in many abseil situations in climbing it's preferable to put as little strain on the anchor as possible.

A few easy practice abseils with a safety rope will equip you with enough knowledge and experience to move on to the next stage, where you abseil without a safety rope. These first practice abseils can be done using a single rope. Out on the cliffs and crags, though, you'll nearly always need to abseil on a doubled rope because the rope will need to be retrieved once each climber has descended. If you climb on a single rope of, say, 60m in length, the maximum distance you're able to abseil is 30m, but if you use double ropes knotted together you can abseil the full length of each rope.

SELF-SAFETY

Once you're happy with the basic techniques, move on to practise using a Prusik knot as a safety back-up. This safety mechanism is what you'll use every time you abseil, so once again it's a good idea to practise in a controlled situation.

There are two scenarios on an abseil where you'll particularly benefit from having a safety back-up mechanism:

- Arresting the descent while you take both hands off the rope to sort out a tangle in the rope or perhaps to retrieve a stuck running belay.
- Accidental injury through falling debris, which might cause you to let go of the controlling rope inadvertently.

The abseil device is rigged in exactly the same way and the safety back-up is attached to the leg loop of the harness or to the abseil loop; the former gives a back-up on the controlling rope and the latter is attached above the abseil device. Experiment with both methods before deciding which you prefer – each has small advantages over the other for particular situations. The method more commonly used is that with the safety back-up attached to the leg loop, via a screwgate karabiner.

The variety of Prusik knot used out of preference is the French Prusik, which is effortlessly released after being subjected to a load as well as being easily slid down the rope as you descend. I don't recommend the use of any other Prusik knot for this purpose, as many of them will jam solid and then can only be released by cutting with a knife.

The length of the Prusik loop is critical: it should be of a length where, once tightened and under load, it doesn't butt up against the abseil device. Ideally the cord used for such a loop should be 110–

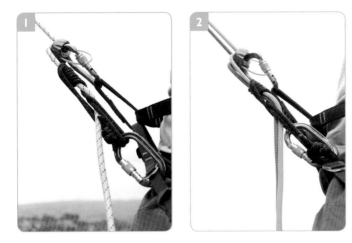

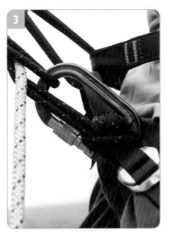

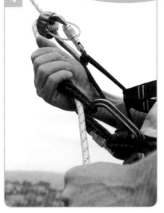

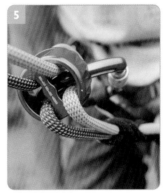

1 When you feel confident at the practice site, try arranging your own safety back-up abseil. Here we see a safety Prusik loop attached below the abseil device and then clipped to the leg loop. There are two small problems with this particular set-up: first, concerning the attachment to the leg loop, the ziplock buckle system has a tendency to slide open when loaded as shown; second, the length of the French Prusik safety comes a little too close to the abseil device (if contact is made the abseil device won't lock automatically).

2 A better way to set up is to use the knotted end of the Prusik loop 'larksfooted' around the harness leg loop; this shortens the overall length of the French Prusik.

3 The detail of the attachment to the leg loop.

4 When descending, keep both hands on the control rope of the abseil below the device. One hand holds the French Prusik and pulls it down as you descend while the other hand controls your speed of descent. With plenty of experience, however, you can use one hand for both purposes.

5 The same set-up used for a double-rope abseil. The safety back-up French Prusik is wrapped around both ropes.

120cm long and of 6mm diameter. If the loop is too long and comes into contact with the abseil device, it won't lock and will therefore be ineffective, causing you to slide ever faster down the abseil rope. If the loop is too short, the turns around the rope may be very tight and prevent smooth descent.

You can also attach the French Prusik above the abseil device, but it's vitally important to ensure that the knot doesn't stretch out of arm's reach when the load is applied. If it does, it'll be difficult to release again. The best gauge for the length of the attachment is for the Prusik to be no more than a slightly bent arm's length from you when the sling becomes tight.

Another form of abseil safety is to hold the bottom of the abseil ropes while someone is descending. If the abseiler loses control during the descent, the person at the bottom should pull the rope very hard. This will halt any further descent until the tension is released. I have seen this used to great effect on a number of occasions that otherwise would have resulted in serious injury.

JOINING TWO ROPES TOGETHER

Though the more usual knot to employ for joining two ropes together is the double fisherman's (or double fisherman's with reef in between), it has become common practice to use a figure of eight or an overhand when joining two ropes for abseiling. If you join the two ropes in this way, when you come to retrieve them after the abseil the knot presents a flatter profile to any edge that it may be dragged over, much reducing the chances of the knot becoming jammed during retrieval.

If you're unfortunate enough to get your ropes jammed, be particularly careful how you go about freeing them. Don't ever, for instance, attempt to climb up a single jammed rope, in case the rope isn't as jammed as it first appears.

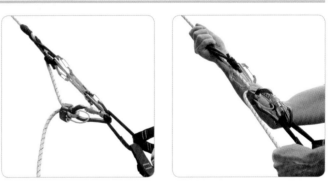

↑ Some climbers prefer to use the safety French Prusik above the device. It's vital to ensure that when the French Prusik is under load you're able to reach the top of it comfortably so that it can be released. Two quickdraws back to back are ideal, but a cowstail attachment would do the same thing. Make sure that you attach to the safety French Prusik with a screwgate karabiner.

↗ To descend, use one hand to control speed and the other to hold the French Prusik slackly on the rope so that it slides down easily.

→ When joining double ropes together, the overhand knot is ideal because it presents a fairly flat profile and makes retrieval of abseil ropes after the descent considerably less problematical. When using this knot, the two ropes must be of equal diameter and you must ensure that there's at least 45cm of spare tail.

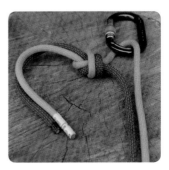

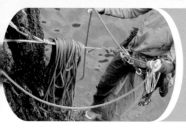
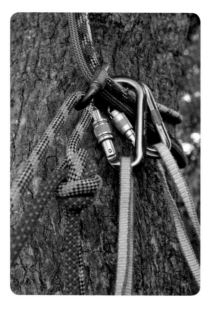

→ This fixed abseil point discourages climbers from securing the rope directly around the tree and damaging its bark. The two screwgate karabiners are the climber's attachment points, via a cowstail; note that in this photo one of the krabs has yet to be screwed shut. The abseil rope is threaded through the maillon to facilitate recovery of the rope after the abseil and, most importantly, to preserve the integrity of the anchor sling by discouraging climbers from threading the abseil rope directly through the sling. A moving nylon rope dragged over a static nylon sling creates sufficient friction to cause the surface of the sling to melt – which will weaken the sling considerably for subsequent users. Attach yourself to the abseil anchor, or a separate anchor, using a cowstail *before* you untie from the end of the rope to thread it through an abseil anchor.

↓ Abseil slings in situ with a corroded screwgate karabiner – this fixed abseil anchor needs to be considered with care. UV degradation is particularly acute on nylon ropes and over a long period can reduce their strength by a high percentage.

↓ This fixed abseil anchor has been in place for a very long time and continually added to by climbers unsure of the level of safety offered by the slings. Ideally all the old rope and tape should be cut away and replaced with new equipment, but unfortunately very few climbers carry sufficient equipment to do this.

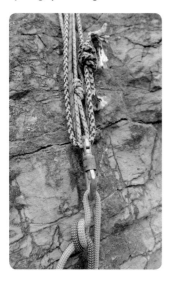

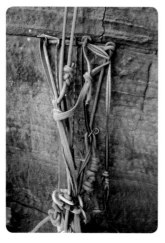

The following sections cover the various forms of abseiling other than the abseil retreat from a climb, which is explained in the next chapter.

DESCENT FROM A FIXED ABSEIL ANCHOR

The accompanying photo shows a tree being used as a fixed abseil anchor at the top of a climb. In this case a rope sling has been permanently fixed around the tree to prevent continual use by climbers from damaging its bark and perhaps causing its eventual death. Similar fixed anchors may be found around rocks.

The maillon is a steel ring that's permanently screwed tightly closed and no attempt should be made to undo it. If you need to do a long abseil, the end of one rope is threaded through and then tied together with the end of the second rope. If half of a single rope is all that's required, then the rope needs to be pulled through the maillon to the halfway mark on the rope.

In some instances you may find that the fixed anchor is made up of several bits of tape or rope slings that may or may not include a maillon or a fixed karabiner – such anchors should be treated with caution. If the rope is threaded directly through a fixed sling, when it's retrieved after the descent the pulling action creates considerable friction, almost certainly generating enough heat to cause a degree of melting of the sling. Past instances of melting, which can often be seen as a hardening of the sling's surface, will weaken the sling and a judgement has to be made as to its safety. A sling that has been in place for a long time will also have been subject to UV degradation, which will not only cause it to fade in colour but also weaken it. If there's any doubt as to the provenance of a sling used as a fixed anchor, it should be replaced or supplemented with a sling of your own.

To set yourself up for an abseil descent from the top of a climb, you first need to untie from the ends of the rope. Before doing this, arrange what's termed a 'cowstail' by using a long sling and attach yourself to the anchor separately from the maillon. Once clipped in, each of you can untie from the ends of the rope or ropes. For an abseil requiring only half of a single rope, thread it through the maillon until the halfway mark on the rope comes into the maillon. For double-rope abseils, thread one end through and join it to the other rope using an appropriate knot. At this point you'll have to make a mental note of which rope you need to pull to retrieve both ropes after the descent; obviously you won't be able to pull the knot through the anchor.

Once threaded and/or tied together, the rope needs to be thrown down the cliff. You'll be abseiling on a doubled rope so each half needs to be thrown separately – and this can present all kinds of issues! If it's windy the ropes may be blown to one side and become caught on a ledge or spike of rock. The cliff may not be steep enough for the ropes to be thrown all the way down. There may be vegetation in which the ropes become entangled. And so it goes on…

There are no golden rules to prevent any of these problems. However, if you throw a short loop of rope down the crag first, starting with the ropes from the anchor, the ends can then be coiled up and thrown down afterwards. Remember to shout 'Rope below!' before launching the ropes off the crag just to warn anyone who might be climbing or walking below.

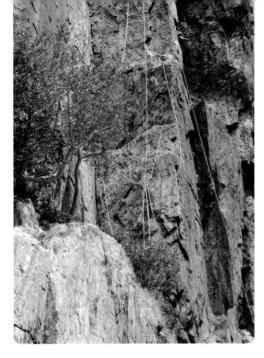

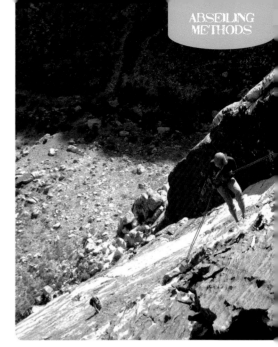

← When you throw abseil ropes down a crag, from time to time they'll become tangled around themselves or amid vegetation. This needs to be sorted out on the descent and you may well have to rely on your safety back-up French Prusik to hold you while you use two hands to sort out the mess.

→ If you're likely to abseil above other climbers who are still ascending, be considerate and warn them that you're throwing ropes down; try to stay out of their way if at all possible.

The first abseiler now attaches to the ropes using a safety back-up Prusik. Once ready to go, quickly check that everything is clipped to the correct points on the harness and all screwgate karabiners are tightened shut, and then, finally, unclip from the cowstail attachment to the anchor.

As the first person descends, any tangles in the rope can be sorted out and two hands can be used if the weight is taken on the back-up Prusik. Never descend below a tangled or jammed rope thinking that it can be sorted by just pulling the ropes down. If you do, the chances are that the rope will remain tangled or jammed and you'll then be faced with the dilemma of climbing back up to free the rope.

Once you're on the ground, shout up to the next climber so that he can get ready to abseil.

MULTIPLE-STAGE ABSEILS

If a single-length abseil doesn't get you back to the ground or on to safe terrain, you'll need to repeat the process.

Whenever an abseil finishes above ground level, tie a knot in the ends of the rope. You can tie separate knots in each end or, preferably, a single overhand knot tied in the two ends. Assuming that a second fixed abseil anchor is in place, the first abseiler down should clip into the anchor using a cowstail before releasing himself from the abseil. Once he's attached to the anchor and detached from the abseil rope, the second abseiler can descend. When both are firmly secured to the anchor, the ropes can be pulled down. As one person pulls the rope the other person can be threading the rope through the maillon on the next abseil anchor. This saves time and minimises the possibility of the ropes being accidentally dropped. Once retrieved, the ropes are then thrown down the cliff and the whole process begins again.

The procedure is slightly different if no fixed abseil points are in place and you have to rig your own to leave behind. The principles of rigging anchors have already been described in previous chapters. The decision that has to be made is what gear to leave behind.

ABSEILING INTO SEA-CLIFF CLIMBS

Climbing sea cliffs is one of the most enjoyable aspects of the sport, though it isn't everyone's cup of tea!

Sea-cliff climbs are accessed in various ways. Sometimes there's just a simple walk to the bottom of the climb at low tide, but this is unusual. Occasionally access is gained by scrambling down to the side

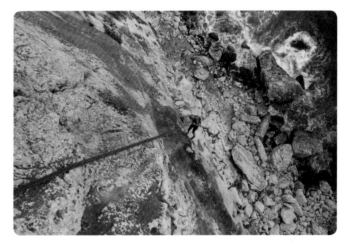

↑ A multiple-stage abseil where the descent utilises the same anchors as those used during the ascent. The climbers used a single 60m rope to climb so the limit of abseil length is 30m. The cowstail that was rigged at the very start of the process remains attached to the harness throughout the descent and is conveniently clipped into the anchor. Always tie a knot in the ends of the abseil rope when the rope doesn't reach the ground.

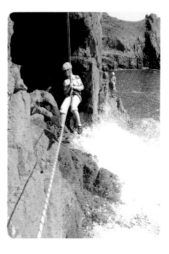

→ Abseiling into climbs above the sea can present all kinds of exciting moments! The last thing you need before beginning a climb is a good soaking, and here the problem is compounded by the fact that the best ledge to belay from is slightly to one side of the line of the abseil. The first climber down has to swing across the face and make an anchor, then the next climber down can abseil to just above the water line and be pulled across by the first climber – this is sometimes called a pendulum.

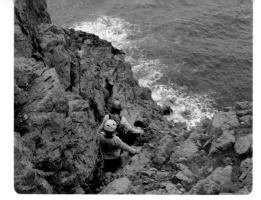

← Some sea cliffs climbs require nothing more than an exposed scramble to reach the bottom.

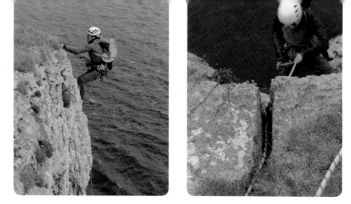

⬆ **When you take the first steps over the edge of a cliff, try to make sure that the abseil rope doesn't run over any particularly sharp edges or get jammed in narrow cracks on the edge.**

of the cliff and then traversing along the foot of the cliff just above the water until you reach the beginning of the chosen route. More often than not, though, an abseil approach will be required, either directly down the climb or off to one side.

In an ideal situation there'll be a large ledge at the base on which you have ample space to sort gear and prepare for the climb. In a less favourable situation you may find that the ledge is tiny or almost non-existent and it will all add up to a big adventure.

At the top of popular sea cliffs you may find existing anchor points, such as metal stakes driven into the ground. While such anchors are most reassuring to discover, they should be treated with circumspect. Salty air corrodes metal quite quickly and unseen rusting and deterioration below ground level may cause weakness.

Many climbers use an entirely separate rope to abseil into sea-cliff

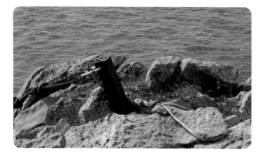

← **Existing anchor points, such as stakes hammered into the ground, need to be treated with suspicion. This is a horrific anchor, but two climbers had descended from it shortly before this photo was taken. The metal stake is rusty and points towards the direction of loading rather than away from it. The attachment with the karabiner is at the highest point, creating leverage on the stake. The attempt to make a back-up anchor to a small flake uses a sling that's way too slack (back-up anchors should be under the same tension as the main anchor so that load is divided equally).**

⬇ **If the abseil anchor is a long way back from the edge of the cliff there could be some stretch in the rope, even when using low-stretch ropes. Here the climbers have sensibly re-anchored to a large flake to take out some of the stretch.**

climbs. Ideally this will be a static or low-stretch rope (usually of 10–11mm diameter) that will be left in place while the climb is undertaken. If you arrive at your chosen descent and discover a rope already in place, it's polite to communicate with the owners of the rope and ask if they mind you using it or if it should be pulled up so that you can use your own rope.

Assuming that you find anchors but no rope, you'll need to rig the anchors so that you can attach an abseil rope. It's better to put your trust in at least two anchors rather than one, even if one alone looks totally solid. With multiple anchors, if one fails the remaining anchor won't be subjected to a shock loading that might result in it failing too. Any anchors you place, including crack protection, should ideally be linked to one central attachment point using the techniques outlined in Chapter 6.

When the end of rope is anchored, throw it down the cliff. If you know for certain that you're going to finish up on a small ledge above the sea, make sure you tie a knot in the end of the rope or ropes, then abseil down the rope making sure that you have a safety back-up Prusik mechanism.

On arriving at sea level you'll need to create an anchor to attach yourself to. Do this before you detach from the abseil completely. Once done you can attach yourself using a cowstail and call for your climbing partner to join you. When you're both at the foot of the climb attached to the anchor, you can begin to sort out and uncoil the ropes you will climb on.

This may prove trickier than expected as it's vital to keep the

⬇ **When you abseil to the beginning of a climb above the sea, or even part way up a cliff, make sure that you create an anchor and attach yourself to it before taking your weight off the abseil rope and detaching yourself from the rope.**

⬇ **Before the start of the abseil the climbing rope was prepared on comfortable, flat terrain, and coiled Alpine-style so that it's easily unwrapped and laid over the ropes to the anchor in laps.**

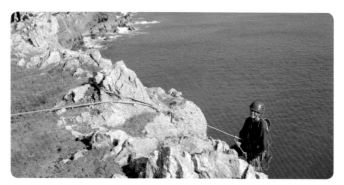

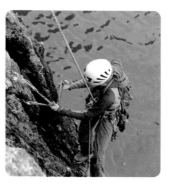

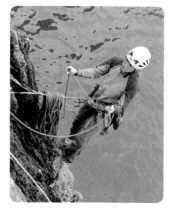

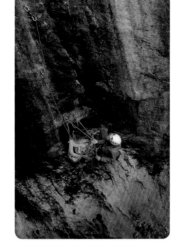

➜ A rope bucket is a great idea for climbing sea cliffs, or indeed in any awkward situation at the start of a climb. You can sort out the ropes at the top of the climb and then abseil with them tidily in the bucket, which is suspended from the belay anchors. Each climber ties on to the correct end of rope: the leader ties to the end at the top of the bucket while the belayer ties to the end at the bottom of it.

ropes out of the water. There may not be sufficient space to put the ropes on a ledge, in which case they'll need to be lapped over the attachment to the anchor itself. A rope bucket (or rope bag) is a great asset when you're on a belay above the sea. You can abseil down with the ropes already uncoiled in the bucket, with the ends of the rope tied to the top loop so they're accessible to both leader and second climber. Alternatively, you can send the belayer down first attached to the climbing rope and as the leader descends the rope can be coiled into the bucket.

It's really important to prepare everything in advance at the top of the cliff so that each of you is aware of what will be required to organise things efficiently. In terms of organising the ropes, you may even consider tying on to them at the top of the cliff. The first climber abseils down with ropes attached ready for climbing while the remaining climber at the top of the cliff allows them to run in unison with the speed of descent. Once the first abseiler reaches the bottom he can rig the anchor and then take in the ropes as the second climber descends, coiling them appropriately to prevent them falling into the sea.

Communication is vital between both climbers: if it's difficult to hear or understand each other's shouted instructions, all sorts of difficulties may arise.

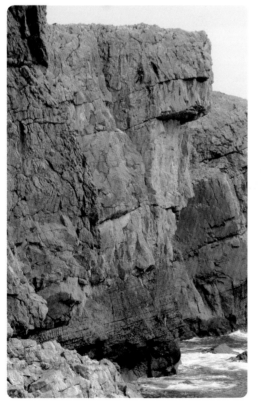

➜ This climb has nothing in the way of ledges at the bottom, so climbers need to abseil down and attach to hanging anchors above the high-water mark.

ABSEILING SAFETY CONSIDERATIONS

Sadly, there have been some tragic abseiling accidents over the years. Though some may reasonably be attributed to fate, others have occurred due to errors of judgement.

Always check the abseil anchor thoroughly. Don't trust old decayed slings or in situ pegs or nuts if you're the slightest bit suspicious of them. It's cheaper to sacrifice a bit of gear rather than a life.

If you know or suspect that the ropes don't reach the ground, a simple but worthwhile safety precaution, such as tying a knot in the ends of the ropes, could prevent a very nasty accident.

To facilitate the separation and recovery of abseil ropes, it's often worthwhile to clip a short quickdraw on to one of the ropes and the other end to your harness. If you do this at the beginning of the descent it will keep the ropes separated all the way to the bottom. Furthermore, if you put it on the rope that you have to pull to retrieve the abseil ropes, it serves as a reminder of the correct rope to pull.

Using two ropes of significantly different diameters can pose serious dangers. For example, a 10.5mm rope used with an 8.8mm rope produces an incompatibility in terms of the friction generated through the abseil device. The thinner rope will run more easily than the thicker rope and a certain amount of rope creep around the anchor will occur. This may in turn lead to unequal lengths of rope hanging down the crag, and if the unsuspecting climber abseils off the end of one rope the whole system will unravel, causing a potentially fatal fall.

If the abseil rope runs over a sharp edge it may cause abrasion of the rope sheath. A scuffed sheath is usually not too much of an issue but if the sheath is actually cut through this presents considerable danger. In a worst-case scenario the sheath may slip all the way along the length of the rope.

If you join two ropes together and retrieval means that they will have to run across a sharply angled ledge when being pulled down, the joining knot may become stuck on the edge, perhaps even embedded in a small crack. If you encounter this potential situation, it can be avoided by ensuring that the knotted join is always over the edge before you descend. This will mean that the rope ends will be of unequal length down the crag so be sure that you're aware of the issue.

Regardless of whether your climbing partner is using a safety back-up Prusik, if you're the first person down try to keep hold of both abseil ropes loosely in your hands. If you see your partner having difficulty, a forceful tug on the rope will prevent him sliding any further down the rope.

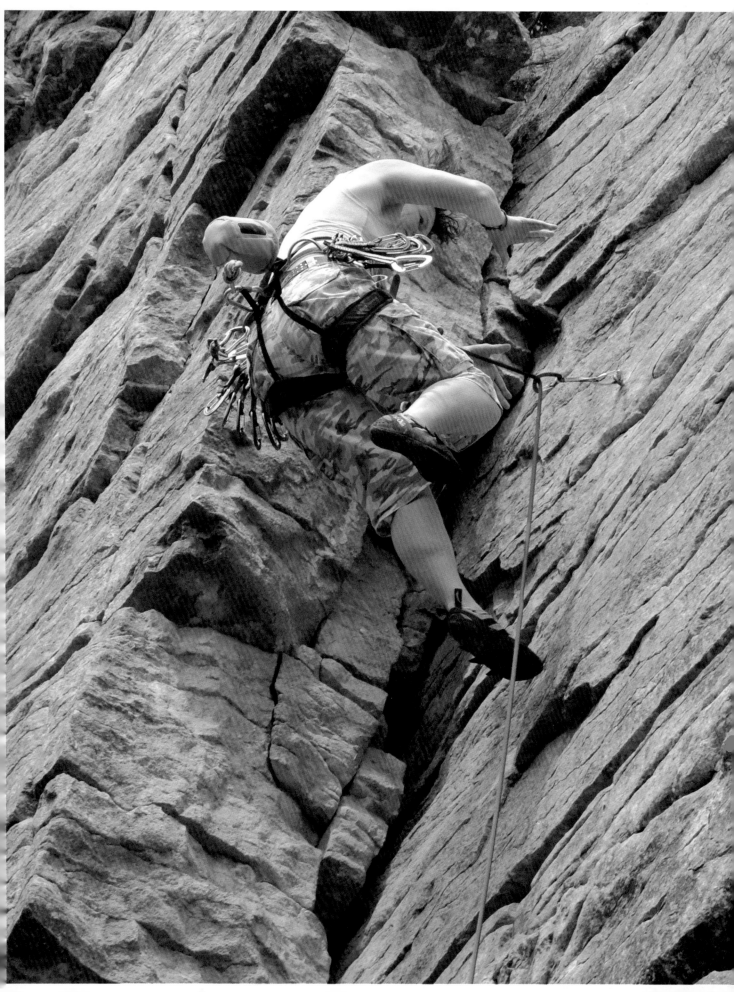

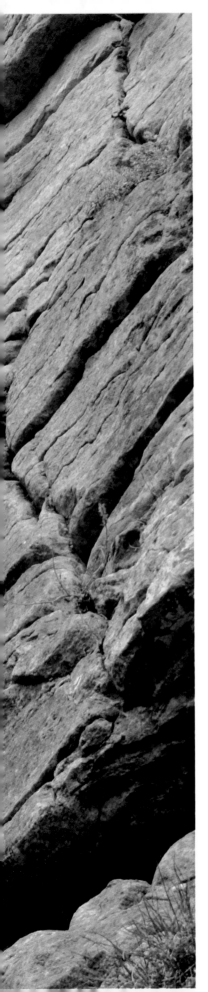

PROBLEM SOLVING

I f you spend a lifetime rock climbing and never get into a tricky
situation or experience some kind of epic, you'll be a very lucky
climber indeed!

Despite your best intentions and attention to safety in every
detail, small things go wrong from time to time, so having the
wherewithal to deal with simple problems should be in every
climber's repertoire of skills. Most solutions to climbing problems
can be dealt with in a relatively simple and straightforward manner
using only the kit that you have at your disposal.

The two most important questions to ask yourself when
presented with a tricky situation are:

- What's the simple solution? And then, just before you embark
  on your solution, pause for a moment to consider the second
  question…
- What will happen if…?

What follows is description of how to deal with some of the
simple problems that may be encountered. Always bear
in mind that the solution to a particular problem
may actually be simpler than the description here.

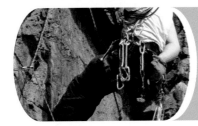

DEALING WITH SIMPLE PROBLEMS

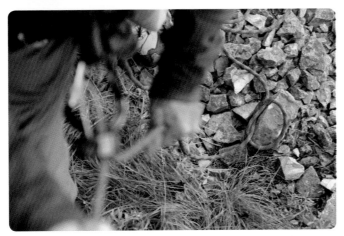

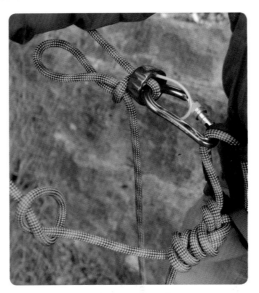

◄→ **A simple knot in the rope can be moved towards the belayer's tie-in point and when the leader is safely anchored it's a simple matter to step through the offending glitch.**

Whenever possible the following techniques should be practised in a controlled situation before you put them to use for real.

A KNOT IN THE ROPE

When you embark on a climb, and at intermediate stances up the climb, you should always make an effort to organise the climbing ropes. By doing so you will know that there are no tangles in the rope and, more importantly, no knots.

Imagine a situation where the leader is part way through a tricky series of moves when the second climber, who's paying out the rope, shouts up, 'Just hang on a minute – there's a knot in the rope.' The leader is likely to have a serious sense-of-humour failure – justifiably.

If you do discover a knot in the rope at an awkward moment, the simplest way to get around the problem temporarily is to move the knot along the rope. When the leader is on a stance or at a part of the climb where he can secure himself comfortably, the knot can then be untied.

If you're climbing on a single rope the knot can be moved along the rope right up to the tie-in point and then 'untied' by stepping through the enlarged, open loops of the knot. If you're climbing using double ropes, you'll almost certainly have to untie from the rope end to undo the offending knot.

Standing on the ground at the foot of the climb is an easier place to deal with a knot in the rope. Being on a small ledge part way up a climb is altogether a different matter and if you have to untie from the end of the rope you'll first need to make sure that you're secured to the rock face by another method. Using a sling as a cowstail is the best way to do this, and is explained later in this chapter.

TYING OFF A BELAY DEVICE

There may be occasions in climbing where you will need to release your control of the climbing ropes while safeguarding a climber. Untying a knot or releasing a tangle in the rope are examples. Another example might be where the leader or second has fallen and is hanging with their full weight on the rope. You may find it more comfortable and certainly more secure to tie off the rope temporarily at the belay device so that you can let go completely with both hands.

⬇ **Twists will develop in the rope from time to time, but quite how this happens is one of climbing's great mysteries! The only way to sort out twists is to untie from the rope and allow them to drop out. Always wait until you're safely anchored on a stance before untying from the rope.**

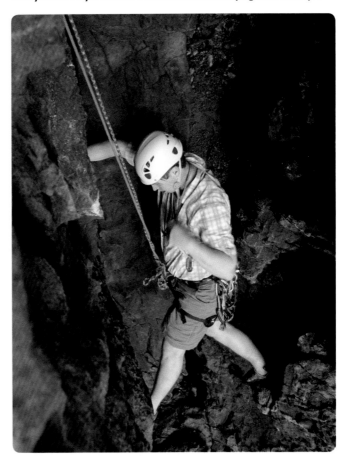

Tying off a belay device

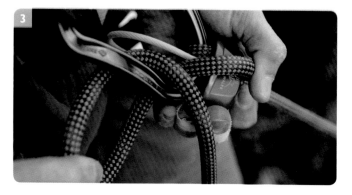

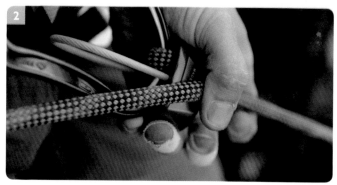

1 Lock the belay device and take the weight of the climber; the right hand is the controlling hand in this sequence.

2 Grip the controlling rope with the whole hand over the belay device and pinch it against the device with the thumb; don't let go of the rope with the controlling hand.

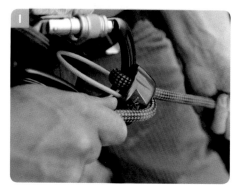

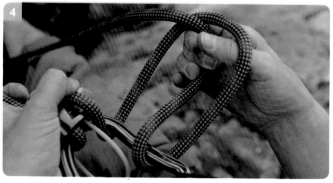

3 Thread the rope through the device karabiner around the back bar of the krab – not the gate. Pull a small loop through.

4 Pull the rope through the loop you've formed.

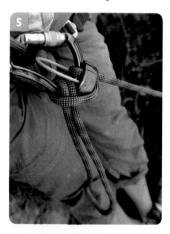

5 Tighten the knot and set it up against the belay device; this should now lock.

6 As a safety back-up, tie a second knot around the back bar of the karabiner.

7 The completed tie-off is totally secure and you can release both hands to sort out any problems.

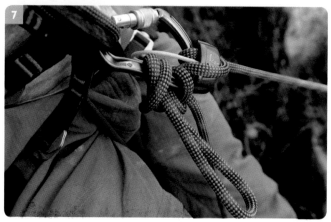

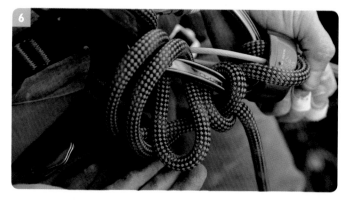

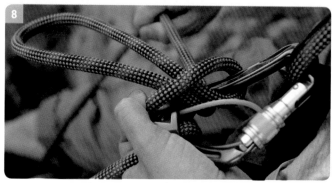

8 To release the tied-off device and get back into climbing or lowering mode, first untie the second knot used as a safety back-up and then grab the device as you did in the second photo. Then all you need to do is pull the rope through the locking loop.

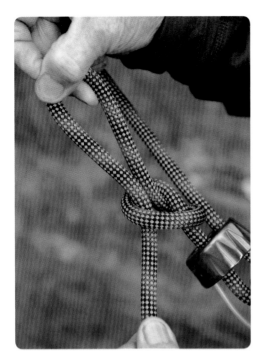

← **To temporarily tie off the belay device you could just tie a simple overhand in the rope up against the device. This is most useful on big ledges where the second will take over the lead. It's a temporary safety measure only and for full security the climber must tie directly to the anchors in the correct way.**

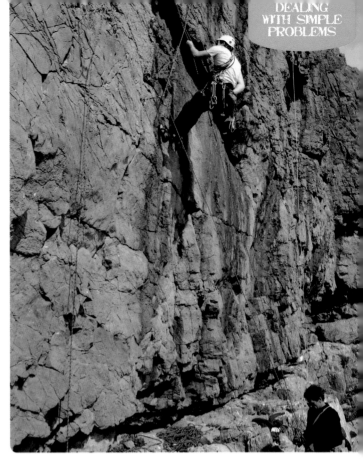

→ **A stuck runner may result from a leader having weighted the placement in order to rest during a difficult move, though it can sometimes be problematical to fathom out how it went in the first instance.**

The accompanying photos show how to tie off a belay device and also how to untie it again to get back into belaying mode. All belay devices of whatever kind can be tied off with the method shown. It's usually much easier to tie off a belay device with weight on the rope but you can also tie it off in the same way without any weight on the rope.

A further photo shows a quick way to temporarily secure the rope, a method that's useful for changeovers on belay ledges when the belayer needs to hand over kit to the climber who will lead the next pitch. It's not suitable for use on small stances where the belay requires the climbers to hang all their weight from the anchors.

RETRIEVING A STUCK RUNNER

Of all the problematical situations that can arise, this is probably the most commonly encountered.

A typical example might be that the second climber has great difficulty extracting a piece of leader-placed protection from a crack. As the leader you may decide to abandon it completely, but if it's an expensive camming device you'll almost certainly want to make some attempt to retrieve it. Before you embark on any complex manoeuvre, ask your second to hang on the rope so that they can use both hands for the task. There'll always be a bit of stretch in the rope so ask the second to climb up above the stuck gear, take the rope really tight and then sit back on it. If you've judged it well your second should be in a good position to hang comfortably and be able to work at releasing the offending gear. You may consider tying off the belay device for extra security.

Usually the problem can be resolved in this way, but, if not, you may decide to go down yourself to have a go. If that's the case, you need to bring the second up to the stance and get him to secure himself to the anchors. Though one option is to arrange an abseil down to try to retrieve the gear, it's probably better to ask your partner to lower you down on the rope or to safeguard you while you climb down. Either way, the second will belay you through his device.

For peace of mind, it's prudent to put on some kind of safety back-up mechanism using a simple French Prusik, as shown in one of the accompanying photos. The auto-locking nature of the French Prusik gives added security to the lowering procedure and if fitted correctly will lock securely if the rope runs a little too quickly for the belayer to control.

Having reached the stuck gear, you can then have a go at retrieving it yourself. Once it has been extracted – or the decision made to abandon it – simply climb back up the route of ascent to the stance. There's no need to remove the French Prusik until you're back at the stance and rearranging everything to continue the ascent.

If there are climbers following you on the same route, you could ask if they would kindly have a go at getting it out. It would be legitimate bounty, of course, so you may have to negotiate a pint or two if they successfully retrieve it!

→ **A French Prusik can be tied around the loaded rope and secured to the same point at which the belay device is attached. To lower a climber (bottom pic) keep a tight grip on the controlling rope in the locked-off position and hold the French Prusik released. If you need to stop, you can allow the French Prusik to grip the rope. Make sure that it holds securely before letting go of the controlling rope and always tie a back-up knot around the karabiner.**

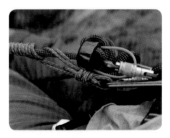

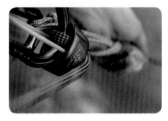

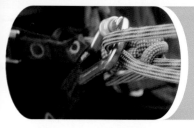

RETREATING FROM A CLIMB

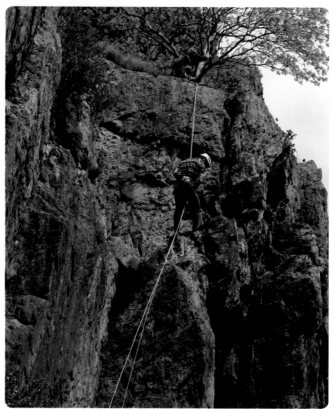

↑ **Retreating from a climb part way up may pose some difficulties.**

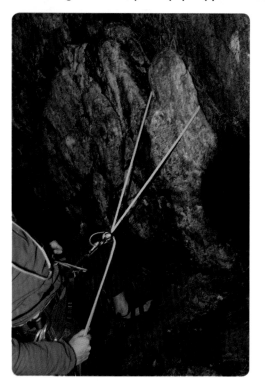

← **When having to retreat from a climb, the ideal feature, though rarely found, is a convenient spike of rock that you can drape the rope around and abseil from, leaving no gear behind at all. You need to be certain that the rope will be retrieved easily and that the flake or spike has no sharp edges.**

There will be occasions in climbing where upward progress comes to a sudden halt. You may be part way up a multi-pitch climb when the heavens open in an almighty downpour, making further progress too difficult and dangerous or just downright unpleasant. You may have chosen a climb that proves too difficult for your ability and experience. Or you may just be having an off day. All climbers experience all of these situations during their climbing careers.

RETREATING FROM THE TOP OF A PITCH

Let's take the simplest scenario, where you and your climbing partner are on a belay ledge three pitches up a multi-pitch trad route when you decide to retreat. You need to abseil off. If the three pitches were quite short and you have double 60m ropes, you may be able to abseil directly to the ground in one go, and let's assume this for now.

First, both climbers need to detach themselves from the climbing rope. Use a cowstail and clip yourself directly to the anchor points before you untie. You also need to decide what you'll use as an anchor to abseil from. Most climbers will be reluctant to leave behind expensive equipment but the priority has to be safety and it's stupid to abseil off marginal anchors for the sake of a few pounds.

The simplest anchor for retreat is a tree, as you can encircle its trunk with the abseil ropes, descend and then retrieve the ropes from the bottom.

The next simplest anchor for retreat is a sling around a flake, provided the flake is solid and without sharp edges where the sling will make contact. All you need do is thread the ropes directly through the sling, tie the ends together and throw the ropes down the crag. When you both reach the ground pull the rope down. This will inevitably cause considerable friction where the rope runs across the sling, but you're down and all you've left behind is a sling that may well be unusable anyway. If you're at all worried about just using a sling, you can sacrifice a karabiner too.

A more expensive option is where crack protection must be left behind. Anchor-construction principles demand more than one piece of crack protection for safety and essentially these principles will apply to the retreat. However, you may decide that one anchor, particularly if it's a bomber nut placement of medium to large size, will be enough. The first climber to descend can go down on this single placement but back it up with another piece of gear or two. In this way the second person to abseil can observe the effectiveness of the single placement without putting the whole team at risk. If all looks good, the last climber to descend will remove the back-up anchors and abseil to the bottom.

If the single anchor you choose is a wire-slung nut, you'll also need to leave a karabiner behind. The angle of bend of the rope directly over a wired nut is too acute for guaranteed safety and in any case will make it incredibly difficult to retrieve the rope once at the foot of the crag. A tape-slung or rope-slung nut is slightly different and you may decide that it's acceptable to thread the rope directly. When and if you decide to leave a karabiner, it need only be a snaplink-gated one, which is less expensive than a screwgate.

The principles of retreating described above can be applied to multiple-abseil descents where one abseil length won't allow you to reach terra firma or you have only a single 50m or 60m rope. It's usual to descend in multiple stages by using the same stances you established on the way up, but bear in mind that you may be able to miss a stance if the length of rope allows, and you should try to ensure that the descent is in as direct a line as possible below the anchors. Obviously, multiple descents will mean that you'll lose more equipment through having to leave gear behind on each abseil.

On any abseil descent where the ends of the rope don't reach the ground, it's sensible to tie a knot in both ends of rope that hang down the crag. This will stop you from accidentally abseiling off the ends of the rope.

RETREATING FROM PART WAY UP A PITCH

There may be occasions where you'll need to retreat from part way up a pitch that you're leading, perhaps because the climb is too difficult or you find yourself off route on something much trickier and need to get back on your correct line.

If it's a difficult pitch that's proving a bit tough, your climbing partner may want to make an attempt at leading the pitch. In this case, simply ask your partner to lower you off the highest running belay back to the belay stance and you can swap responsibilities. The new leader sets off to try climbing the pitch and, if successful, all's well and you can continue with the climb.

If your partner doesn't fancy having a go, you'll need to retreat. This is most simply effected by lowering off the highest runner placement, retrieving all the gear below as you're lowered off, and finally, once you've secured yourself to the ledge, untying from the rope end and pulling it back through the top runner.

The only major decision you'll have to make is whether or not you're happy to put all your faith in a single running belay. If you're not, leave a couple of runners behind. Whatever you decide, you must leave behind a karabiner through which the rope runs. You must never run the risk of lowering off with the rope running through a nylon sling or directly around the wire of a wire-slung nut. If you're on a sports climb and need to lower off, you could just leave behind a single karabiner.

Of course, if you find yourself unable to continue with the climb having retreated from a pitch, you'll then need to continue the retreat by abseil.

ASSISTED HOIST

Any climbing emergency that requires hoisting a climber up the crag should be avoided if at all possible. The exception to this basic premise is where the second climber is having considerable difficulty overcoming a particular section; if this is the hardest part of the climb and the subsequent pitches are easier, you might consider an assisted hoist.

An assisted hoist can only be successfully implemented given a certain number of pre-conditions, the three most important of which are:

- The climber is more or less directly below you.
- The climber is close enough below that you still have, at the absolute minimum, two thirds of the length of spare rope available to you.
- The climber must be in a fit state to help.

The solution is simple enough. Tie off the belay device. Take up some coils of the rope that you have on the ledge beside you and drop a double loop down to your climbing partner. Ask him to clip this loop via a screwgate karabiner directly to the belay loop of his harness. While the climber is doing this, rig up a French Prusik safety back-up.

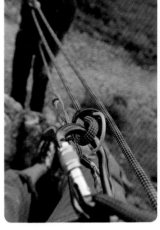

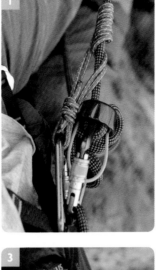

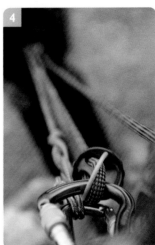

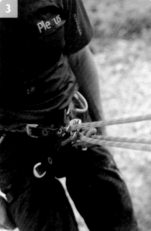

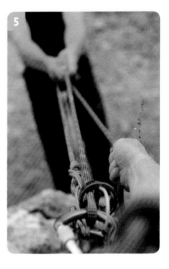

Assisted hoist procedure

1 **Tie off the belay device and attach a French Prusik to the same points where the belay device is attached.**

2 **Preferably before you release the tied-off belay device, throw down to the second climber a loop of spare rope with a screwgate karabiner attached.**

3 **Ask the second climber to clip the karabiner into the belay loop of his harness.**

4 **You now have a pulley system – make sure it's set up without any twists.**

5 **The second pulls up on the middle rope at the same time as the belayer pulls up on the slack rope. The main tie-in or 'live' rope should run smoothly through the device and the French Prusik will automatically release itself. If you both need to rest, make sure that the French Prusik is gripping the rope securely before slackening your hold on the ropes.**

on the 'live' rope and connect it with a separate screwgate karabiner either to your own harness belay loop or to the tie-in rope loop. When these actions have been completed, release the tied-off belay device and pull through any slack rope that develops.

You now must work together. The stuck climber pulls on the 'dead' rope from the belay device and you, as the belayer, pull on the rope that forms the original loop you threw down to your partner. If you both pull at the same time, the arrangement works as an efficient pulley system where the load is shared equally between the two of you and the French Prusik acts as a safety back-up by locking on to the rope when you both need to rest. Once you're both back together on the belay stance you can sort out the mess of ropes and get back into climbing mode.

This self-help technique will require a fair amount of practice before you can be confident of implementing it on a crag for real. To begin with you should try it out on a steep grassy bank where you have plenty of margin of safety.

ASCENDING A ROPE

In Chapter 4 we looked at knots that can be used for ascending a fixed rope or as safety back-ups, but without going into detail of how they might be used.

You could comfortably spend a lifetime climbing without having to ascend a rope as an emergency 'get-out-of-jail' solution to a problem. If you climb on sea cliffs, or any cliff reached by abseil, and you get into difficulties with the climb, the only way out might be to ascend the rope that you used to abseil in the first instance.

Another scenario might be one where you inadvertently abseiled too far beyond a suitable stopping point on a multiple-abseil descent. Such occurrences are very rare, but it's good to be prepared for that 'just-in-case' moment.

Ascending a fixed rope in itself is relatively straightforward but it requires a considerable amount of energy.

The basic set-up necessitates two Prusik loops. One is attached to the harness belay loop and the other is used for a foot loop. The efficiency by which you can measure success is determined largely by how high you can step up in the foot loop. The most efficient way is to use quite a short foot loop that will allow you to make as high a step as is physically possible.

The procedure begins with taking all of your weight on the Prusik loop attached to the harness. If you're attempting to ascend a climbing rope, there'll be an inordinate amount of stretch in the rope to be taken up before you even begin the ascent. A static abseil rope will be more instantaneous though there'll still be some stretch to take up. Once all the stretch has been taken out and you're hanging entirely from the sit loop, put the foot loop Prusik on below the sit loop.

It's better to use one foot in this loop and, as one leg tires, swap to the other. Slide the foot loop as high as is comfortable, cock your foot under your backside and, using hands on the rope to pull, step up simultaneously. Once standing, slide the sit loop up until you can comfortably sag all your weight back on to it and take a rest. Repeat several hundred times until you're on safe ground!

Every two metres or so, tie a figure of eight knot in the rope below the foot loop and clip it to your harness belay loop. This is a good safety mechanism if the sit loop Prusik fails for whatever reason.

The illustrations show the standard Prusik knot being used for both

Ascending a fixed rope using Prusik loops

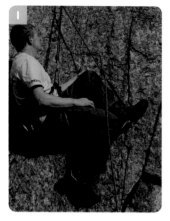

1 **A basic set-up for ascending a fixed rope using Prusik loops. A short foot loop means that greater height can be gained with each sequence but it's largely dependent on how high you can step up. It's possible to extend the foot loop using a sling. You could also set up the system with a foot loop above the sit loop but it'll need to be much longer. Make sure that any knot can be reached comfortably when loaded.**

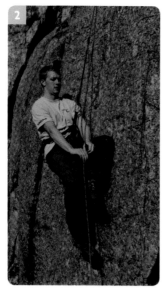

2 **To start to ascend, sit back with all your weight on the sit loop, slacken the foot loop Prusik knot and slide it as high up as is comfortable.**

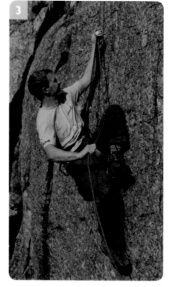

3 **Step up, using a combination of powerful leg muscles and pulling up with one hand. It's easier to grip the knot to help pull yourself up – this is why the sit loop should never be attached with a French Prusik as it will release when you pull it.**

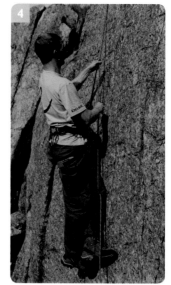

4 **Stand up straight and move the sit loop Prusik up, then immediately sag your weight back on to the Prusik loop to rest. Repeat until you reach safety.**

→ **Periodically on a long ascent, tie a safety back-up knot in the rope and clip it to the belay loop of the harness.**

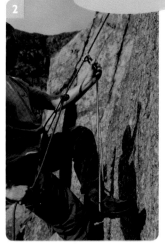

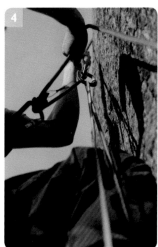

loops, but it isn't essential to use this. You could equally use a Klemheist or even a French Prusik, though with the latter you must be careful not to accidentally pull down on top of the knot while it's loaded as it will release.

Many climbers carry one Prusik loop, which can be used effectively for abseil safety too, and a rather natty device called a Ropeman. Light in weight but super-efficient, this is a mechanical device for ascending a fixed rope. The suggested set-up for a Ropeman is the opposite way round to using loops: attach the Ropeman to your harness belay loop directly with a screwgate karabiner but use the foot loop above the Ropeman; as you stand up in the foot loop, the slack rope can be pulled easily through the Ropeman and sitting back to rest is effected immediately.

Another useful and efficient device that can be used instead of a Prusik loop is the Tibloc. This, like the Ropeman, has multiple uses in the wider sphere of mountaineering as well as for rock climbing.

Don't forget that you can also use a thin tape sling as a Prusik loop; just note that the Klemheist is the most efficient knot to ascend the rope with a sling.

LOWERING YOUR CLIMBING PARTNER

There may be occasions when it's preferable to lower your climbing partner rather than abseil. An example might be where the climber has failed to follow a pitch and it's simpler to lower him back to the ground or to the previous belay stance. Another example might be where it's difficult to throw ropes down the crag to carry out an abseil descent. Having lowered your partner you can then abseil down and join him to continue with the descent.

It's possible to lower a climber from within the system, in much the same way as you might lower on a sports climb or indoor wall lower-off. The significant difference here, though, is that the full weight of the climber must be taken directly on to the harness or, if possible, shared between yourself and the attachment to the anchor.

It's important not to underestimate how tricky it is to lower someone directly off your harness, particularly if the person is quite heavy. Any misalignment of the attachment to the anchor in relation to the direction of the load will be amplified, so make sure that everything is in a straight line. As a precaution you should really use a safety back-up mechanism in the form of a French Prusik auto lock.

Make sure that the rope you need to feed out is stacked neatly on the ledge by your side and that the climber who's being lowered is aware that all of his body weight should remain on the rope throughout the lower.

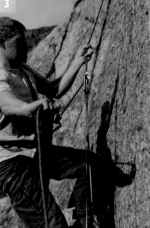

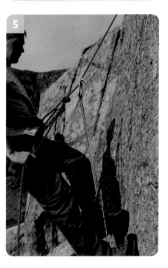

Ascending a fixed rope using a mechanical device

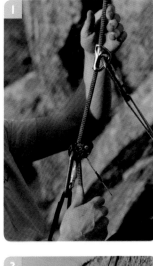

I **This is the set-up for using a mechanical device: Tibloc or Ropeman. Either of these can be used instead of – or in combination with – a Prusik loop. Always attach using screwgate karabiners.**

2 **Move the foot loop up the rope. The mechanical device is released by sliding the karabiner up into the wider part of the slot; it can then be pushed up easily.**

3 **As you stand up, the rope can be pulled through the mechanical device.**

4 **The efficiency with which the rope can be pulled through the mechanical device makes it ideal for attaching directly to the sit loop of the harness.**

5 **Stand up straight in the foot loop and sag back on to the mechanical device for a rest.**

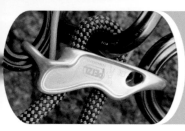

DIRECT BELAYS

A direct belay is the term used to describe a situation where the belay device is connected directly to an anchor point and any load is taken directly on the anchor itself. To use anchors directly in this way you have to be 100 per cent certain that you have sound anchors. Any anchor failure will be catastrophic.

Direct belays are *never* used to safeguard a lead climber. The most appropriate situations when you might elect to use a direct belay are:

■ On easy ground in between pitches on a climb. It's important to assess the level of difficulty of the section of ascent before deciding to use a direct belay. Where it's very simple to scramble

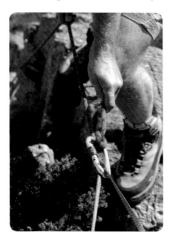

← **A direct belay using an Italian hitch attached directly via a sling to the anchor; remember always to use a rounded-end screwgate karabiner for the hitch.**

⬇ **The Petzl Reverso 4, like the Black Diamond ATC Pro, can be used, attached directly to an anchor, in order to bring up a second climber. Set up as shown, the rope can be pulled through the device but when loaded it will lock solid (the rope running off to the right is direct to the climber and the vertical rope the control rope). If you have the climber's weight hanging on the device, it can only be released by clipping a small karabiner into the small hole on the under-edge of the device. By levering the karabiner upwards the rope will begin to slide through. When you release the device in this way you must always keep a firm grip on the controlling rope.**

up, the leader will climb up, arrange an anchor and then bring the second up on the rope using either an Italian hitch or maybe a particular kind of belay device such as a Petzl Reverso 4 or the Black Diamond ATC Pro. This system of belaying is based on a very old device known as the 'Magic Plate', which has tended to become the generic term for using a belay device in this way. Not all belay devices are suitable for this technique.

■ Descending from a climb where there may be some exposed or slightly tricky section of down climbing and one climber feels the need for some added security from the rope. A simple sling around a flake anchor and an Italian hitch on an HMS karabiner will provide that extra little bit of comfort. Sometimes you may find that you can drape the rope directly around a flake and safeguard the climber in this way.

You may also choose to lower your companion down the cliff. Once again you can use an Italian hitch or you could tie yourself into an anchor and belay normally, as you might do on a climb, but this is a rather more long-winded set-up. You could use a belay device directly attached to the anchor but note that to use a belay device correctly you have to stand and operate it from behind, otherwise it won't lock or create sufficient friction to control the speed of lower. A safety back-up French Prusik is essential!

The speed at which a climber is lowered is dependent on a number of factors. One is how comfortable the climber is about being lowered: if you're more familiar with abseil descents where speed is controlled by your own grip on the rope, having someone else do it is slightly alarming at first. Rate of descent is also determined by the complexities of the terrain: it's all very straightforward if the way down is over an open slab of relatively low angle, but if there are overhangs to negotiate or ledges to pass it can upset the rhythm of descent. Be sympathetic when lowering – that's the key thing.

⬇ **A direct belay is where the rope is used directly around the anchor or attached via a sling with screwgate karabiner and Italian Hitch. All of the load will come on to the anchor so you have to be certain that it's solid.**

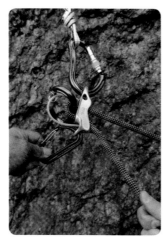

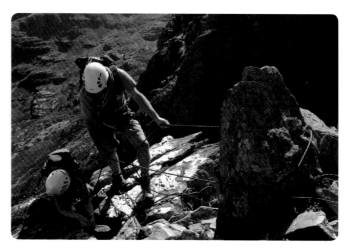

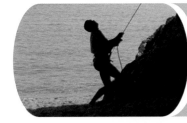
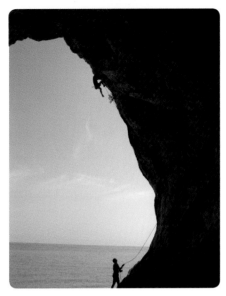

Holding a falling leader

⬆ The belayer is attentive to the leader.

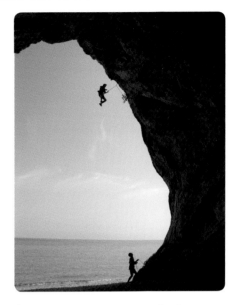

⬆ The belayer is in the process of paying out rope when he spots that the leader is about to fall. There's plenty of rope out between the two as the leader was way beyond the protection, and there's very little time to react.

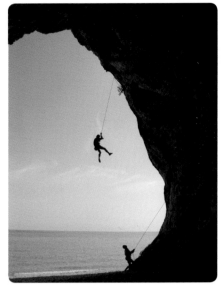

⬆ The belayer must lock off the belay device and be ready to absorb the force of the fall. The amount of rope out and the stretch in the whole system are the shock-absorbing properties ('dynamic' belay).

Having to hold a falling leader is both an emergency procedure and also par for the course, so to speak, particularly as you progress through the grades and climb harder on sport routes.

It's very rare for a leader to fall totally unexpectedly. Usually the only time that it's likely to occur is if a handhold suddenly snaps or a foot slips off and the climber is unable to hold himself at the moment it occurs. If this happens, the distance a leader falls will depend entirely on how vigilant the belayer is at the time, how much slack rope there is in the system and, of course, whether the running belays hold in the rock. This can rightfully be considered an emergency but hopefully the outcome won't be too serious.

Situations in which you might expect a leader to take a fall include the following:

◼ At an indoor climbing wall or outdoor sport route where the leader is attempting something that's quite difficult, maybe at the limit or beyond their climbing ability.
◼ Outdoors on a trad climb that's really difficult (and probably way beyond the scope of most readers of this book).

A leader fall in these situations could be anything from a slump on to the rope with a running belay close to the tie-in point or a massive 'whipper' fall of several metres.

The first thing to consider if you're likely to need to hold a leader fall is the type of belay device you use. Slotted belay devices work superbly well but there's absolutely no margin for error in holding the fall. If you have a loose grip on the controlling rope at the moment of loading, it could very easily get wrenched from your grasp and there'll

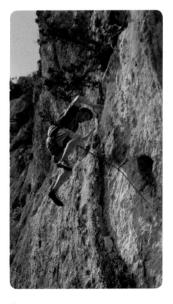

⬆ Here the leader has warned the belayer that he's going to jump off, so there are no surprises. As the rock is slightly overhanging, there's nothing in the way below him.

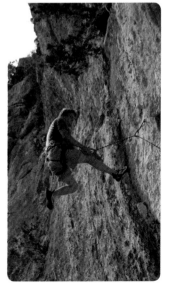

⬆ In the expectation of slamming back into the rock, the falling leader pushes his legs out ready. It's vital to keep the rope in front or to one side if you fall as a leader. If it should get caught between your legs, the moment the load comes on to your harness you will flip upside-down.

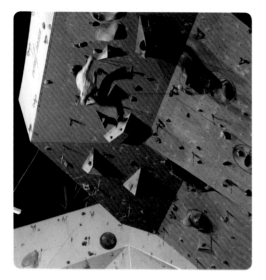

An indoor climbing wall is a good place to practise holding leader falls. Just make sure that small falls are taken initially and that the belayer has a back-up person to hold the controlling rope.

With a short fall on rock that's not particularly steep, you must be attentive to the possibility of injury. Sometimes you may wish to push yourself out a little so that the fall is not a sliding fall.

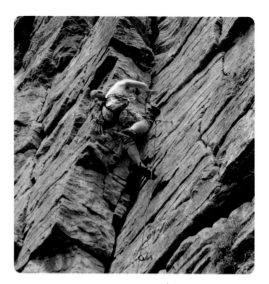

be no way to get hold of it again. The attention of the belayer mustn't slacken at any time. Devices such as the Click Up, GriGri or Edelrid Eddy are ideally suited to these situations as there's an element of auto-locking in their design, though you must never release your hold on the controlling rope at any time.

The other thing to consider when holding a fall concerns the forces exerted on the whole safety system, including the bodies of the climbers themselves. In a fall where the leader simply slumps on to the rope, there's very little force above and beyond the climber's weight. However, a fall of two or three metres will generate considerable force that running belays, bodies and belay device must absorb – no part of the system can be allowed to fail.

The preference for belayer and lead climber is to employ a dynamic style of belaying in which any forces generated are absorbed gradually before the falling leader comes to a final halt. In fact, within the safety system there's reasonable capacity to absorb the force without introducing more, as the stretch in the rope and the climbers' bodies themselves are the two main shock-absorbing devices, while harnesses and knots will also absorb force. Even so, in the few milliseconds it takes from falling off to arresting the fall, none of this will be readily apparent to either belayer or leader until both come to the realisation that the fall was actually further than expected!

There are times when it may be advantageous to deliberately allow the fall to be longer than it might otherwise be, thereby increasing the dynamic element of arresting the fall. This is more applicable to falls on to trad-placed crack protection, but can equally apply to outdoor sport climbing where bolt protection is quite widely spaced.

Before going any further with this, it's worth mentioning that not all climbs are particularly accommodating for falling leaders. Any fall where the leader slides down the rock or catches a foot on an obstacle is very unwelcome, whereas a fall on overhanging rock, where the leader will only fly through the air, is less likely to cause injury.

I've heard climbers talk of allowing rope to slip through the belay device to gradually slow down a falling leader. This is a complete fallacy and, worse, a very dangerous tactic. A fall happens so quickly that there's very little time to think about anything else but arresting it. In any case, semi-auto-locking belay devices won't allow this.

The right way to gradually slow down a falling leader is to stand a little way out from the base of the climb and, as you feel the load coming on to the rope, move towards the base a little or allow yourself to be pulled inwards by the force generated by the falling

leader. Of course, this technique has limited value if you're confined to a small ledge part way up a multi-pitch sport or trad climb.

Holding a falling leader requires a good deal of practice before you can expect to fully appreciate the necessary techniques. Indeed, as a leader it's also a good idea to practise taking a fall. As I've said before, indoor climbing walls are great places to practise in safety. Always make sure that the belayer has a back-up person to hold the controlling ropes for extra safety. Begin with small slumps on to the rope and gradually build up the length of fall taken. Don't ever move on to longer falls until you're comfortable with every aspect of a shorter one.

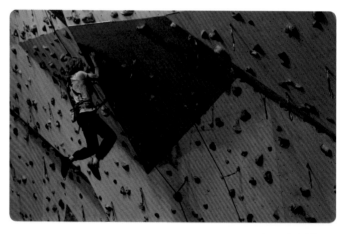

The belayer must remain attentive at all times: very often there are unspoken warning signs that a fall may be imminent.

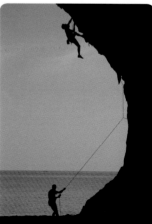

A slump on to the rope with a runner above; the belayer can move backwards from the base of the crag in order to take the rope tighter.

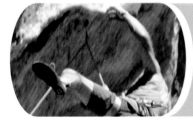

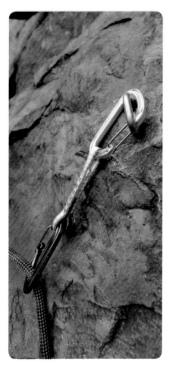 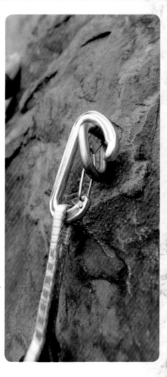

⬆⬈ **The consequences of a karabiner unclipping itself from a bolt accidentally are too horrendous to contemplate. These two images show how it might happen. The karabiner sits on the top of the bolt and a twisting action opens the gate. At this point the krab would simply fall off the top of the bolt.**

➡ **I'd never witnessed this phenomena until looking through some of the shots taken for this book and noticed this. Fortunately it came to nought and as the climber moved up the krab swung back into the correct position.**

There have been occasions when quickdraws have mysteriously unclipped themselves from bolts. It's a very unusual occurrence but one that you should be aware of. It seems that it can only happen with a particular style or shape of bolt hangar. It can happen when the karabiner attached to the bolt accidentally loops itself on to the top of the bolt. The accompanying photos show the position the krab needs to be in to prevent this potentially serious situation.

There are many other tricky climbing situations that you may have to deal with. The simple solutions offered here will work for most of them but as you progress and gain experience, perhaps on bigger faces in remote places, you may well encounter all manner of difficulties and even situations demanding a retreat with an injured companion. These are complex to solve and require a far higher level of knowledge and experience to overcome.

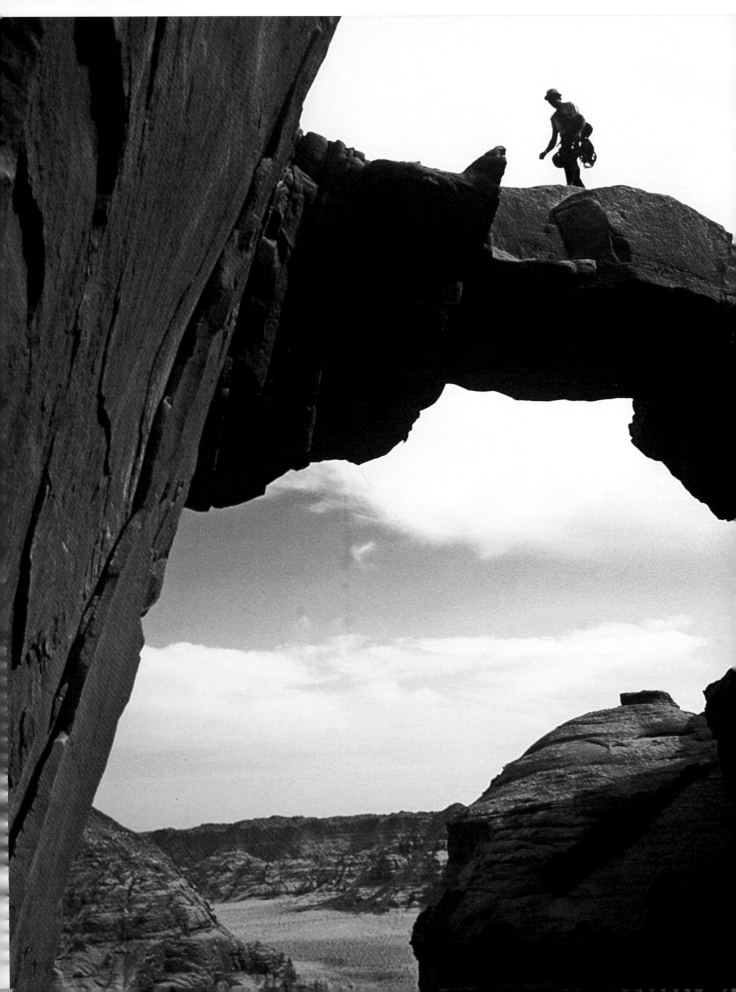

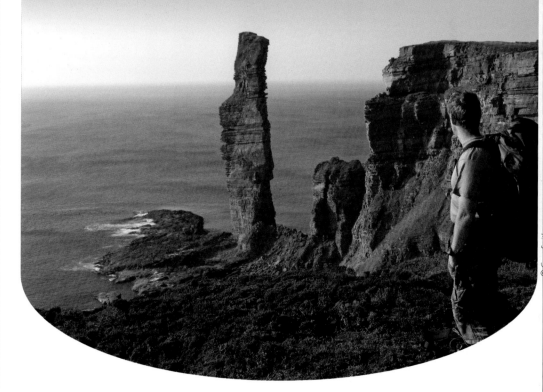

CHAPTER 10
MOVING ON

As you gain confidence and experience both with your climbing technique and handling all the paraphernalia and knots associated with rock climbing, it's perfectly natural to want to push yourself a little and to explore more difficult and more serious climbs. The days of long drawn-out climbing apprenticeships when it used to take years and years to progress through the grades are long gone – though there are those who lament the loss of this rite of passage!

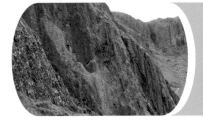

PROGRESSING THROUGH THE GRADES

There are distinct advantages in not pushing hard too early on. Rock climbing has so many different aspects to it that competencies usually only mature after considerable experience. A good way to try harder climbs is with a competent technical climber who has climbed for years and can take care of the safety aspects with great skill and consideration.

Alternatively you may decide that climbing with a qualified instructor or mountain guide is preferable. This is particularly relevant if you don't know anyone who has the necessary experience to lead you up harder climbs. It's even possible to hire a professional for a particular project you might have in mind. I was once hired to climb Left Wall on Dinas Gromlech in North Wales, a steep and strenuous E3 5c. When we met up the gentleman told me that he only needed me to hold his ropes while he led the climb! He did this with ease and we then climbed four other extreme routes on the same crag that day.

An indoor climbing wall is a great place to push up your climbing standard, on the lead particularly. Many climbers progress incredibly quickly indoors to achieve quite high standards in a very short time, given a certain level of natural strength and agility. Unfortunately this doesn't always translate to real climbs in the outdoors. Many climbers find this slightly perplexing but the reasons are simple enough. If you frequent one or two particular climbing walls you'll learn very quickly the style of holds there and what each differently shaped hold has to offer in terms of handhold or foothold. Climbing walls also rely on experienced climbers to set routes and each route-setter has a penchant for particular styles. These two facts combine to make indoor climbs fairly predictable and therefore simpler undertakings.

Real rock has almost infinite variety. Handholds and footholds are rarely the same and seldom in the most ideal position for sequencing moves. Add to that the unknown nature of protection for the leader and you have a far more challenging situation on your hands.

Sport climbing is a very good way to improve your standard. You usually have the comfort of well-spaced, solid protection and also the great variety of handholds and footholds that real rock offers.

Pushing your grade on trad climbs is another dimension. Where once, as a beginner, you stood comfortably on large footholds, able to take both hands off the rock to place 'bomber' protection, harder trad climbs are alarmingly less amenable in this respect. Not only may you find yourself hanging on with one hand to holds of seemingly ever-decreasing size, but also the gear placements may become slightly more marginal and with fewer opportunities for placements. Tiny, wired nuts may be required to gain even the slightest of comfort and you may be confronted with the dilemma of making sequences of moves well above placed running belays.

All this conspires to mess with the physiological elements of climbing, where your mind begins to play games that your body won't listen to or, conversely, your body plays tricks that your mind can't quite understand. Keeping a cool head is an important attitude to nurture in order to progress.

⬅ **In order to push yourself to climb harder grades you'll need to train and to climb aplenty – you won't be this ripped without some dedication.**

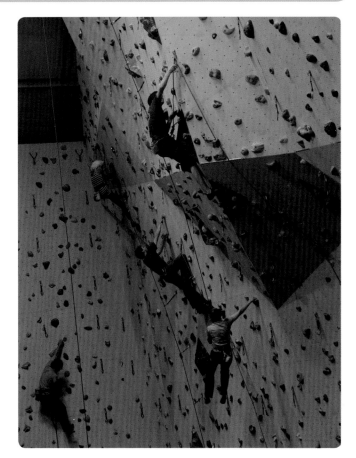

⬆ **An indoor wall with an extensive bouldering area is an excellent place to develop skill, strength and power. The greatest advantage is that you can continue to climb and train unaffected by weather.**

⬇ **The appropriately named Suicide Wall in North Wales. Pushing your standard of climbing on trad climbs where protection is sparse requires a high level of mental control in addition to climbing skills and the ability to arrange protection. Climbs such as this, Capital Punishment E4, are usually only attempted after a long apprenticeship.**

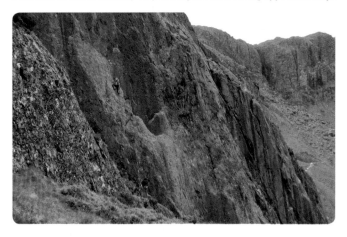

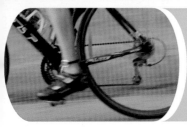

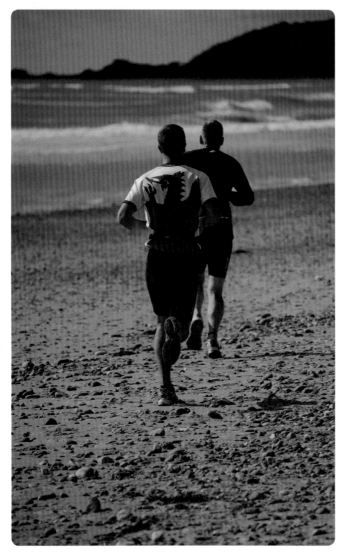

A training regime for rock climbing pays dividends much as it does with many other high-energy and powerful sports. Many indoor climbing facilities offer training programmes, as do independent agencies. Most training for climbing will be centred on three elements:

■ **Physical fitness** – mainly cardiovascular. Activities such as running or cycling are ideal and will help develop the body's ability to recover after periods of more intense activity.

■ **Overall strength** – the stronger you are the more confidently and better you will climb. This is particularly important on short but extremely strenuous climbs where overall physical fitness alone is insufficient for success and where good technique may be an advantage but not necessarily a precursor to success. To train for strength, you must train specific groups of muscles that do different things in climbing. For example, finger and lower-arm strength are important muscle groups for hanging on to tiny crimps but biceps and shoulder muscles are used mainly for hanging on to 'juggy' holds on overhanging rock. An effective training regime for finger strength might be hanging by your fingers from a campus board or similar and for upper arm and shoulder strength pull-ups are a good exercise. Any form of strength training should be undertaken with fresh or rested muscles both to be effective and to reduce the risk of injury.

■ **Endurance strength** – climbing requires considerable levels of endurance strength as well as moments of explosive strength. A long section of sustained climbing at a high level of difficulty will sap power rapidly. The best way to develop power endurance is to train at a level where you're pretty much at the limit of being able to hold on (climbers call this being 'pumped') and then keep going until you can barely hold anything.

It's vital to avoid injury while training for climbing. Strained or torn muscles or tendons can take considerable time to heal, leaving you out of action for weeks or even months. Stretches and warm-ups before strenuous activity will help get the body moving, and going straight on to a strenuous or 'fingery' style of climb on an indoor wall could wreak untold damage. An ideal warm-up is some kind of aerobic exercise followed by stretching and then some easy climbing hanging on to big holds.

As with training for any sport, training for climbing requires a structured regime to be effective.

↑↓↘ **A high level of aerobic fitness is essential: sports such as running, mountain biking and road cycling are all excellent activities to get your heart and lungs working.**

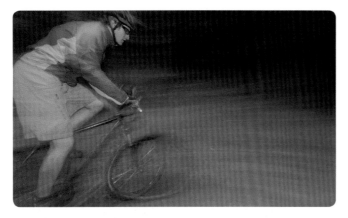

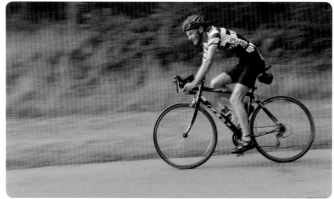

→ **Whether you climb at a low level of difficulty or at the hardest grades, sometimes your mind plays tricks on you and conspires to create a rather discomforting experience. To a certain extent you can learn to control your emotions of fear and apprehension and develop more positive thoughts.**

TRAINING YOUR MIND

In his excellent book *9 out 10 climbers make the same mistakes*, Dave MacLeod, one of the UK's strongest and most talented climbers, cites irrational fear as one of the most significant factors holding back a climber's personal progress.

Fear is a good thing in climbing. It's the primary safety factor that'll keep you safe and well, not allowing you to push too far into the realms of danger. Irrational fear is largely centred around fear of failure and fear of falling, and to a certain extent can be controlled.

If you're a strong and talented climber, experienced and supremely fit, you'll almost certainly have total belief in your ability to climb rock of almost any level of difficulty. In this state irrational fear is pretty much non-existent. But not all of us have this capacity of total belief and even those who do will have days where doubt can creep in. As a mere mortal climber, it's possible to train yourself to focus on controlling irrational fears, such as falling.

Indoor climbing walls are a great place to start. Don't go for a big 'whipper' fall immediately. Begin with short sags on to the rope and gradually increase them in length until you feel comfortable. Obviously falls should be taken well above the floor and preferably on slightly overhanging terrain where you're less likely to hit objects on the way down.

Don't jump off, as doing so may push you further out from the wall and you'll probably crash back into the wall as you come to a halt. Simply let go. Grabbing hold of the rope just above the tie-in knot will help to keep you upright and you need to be alert enough to absorb the shock of hitting the wall with your feet and legs.

One tactic that seems to work really well is to climb a route and when you reach the top, where you would normally clip the rope in to lower off, just fall off instead. Start gradually and build up to longer falls as you gain confidence.

Needless to say, your belayer must be totally competent to hold a fall and this in turn can be really good belaying practice as you begin to appreciate the forces involved in a leader fall.

BOULDERING

Bouldering indoors and outdoors is great training. Before the advent of indoor climbing walls and bouldering mats, this was mostly how climbers trained. Today bouldering is very much a sport in its own right and many climbers just boulder. It can be a sociable activity shared with friends or something that can be done alone amid the tranquillity of the hills. Coincidentally it's great exercise and a fantastic way to develop the technique and skills required to work out sequences of moves.

Boulder problems take many forms. There are those that begin sitting on the ground and may comprise only two or three moves, while there are others that border on being 'micro' rock climbs and finish alarmingly high off the ground. These higher boulder problems are called 'highballs' and they require a studious spotter and, depending on the landing if you were to fall off, several bouldering mats.

Bouldering is all about pure movement over the rock, free of the accoutrements of sport climbing or trad climbing, and without the need to know all manner of fancy rope tricks. For many, this purity is the greatest attraction.

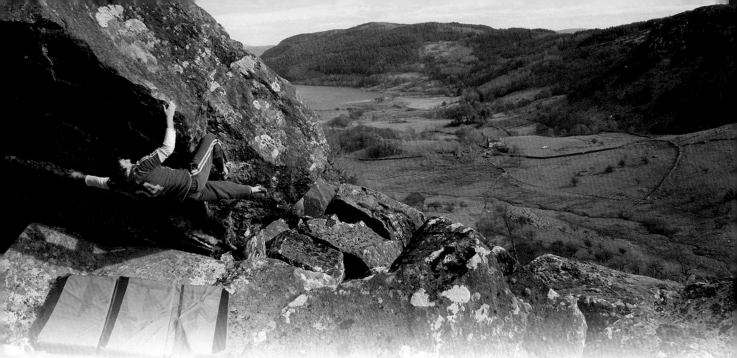

⬆ **Grasswind 7c in the beautiful, peaceful Crafnant valley, North Wales.**
(© Simon Panton)

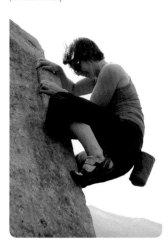

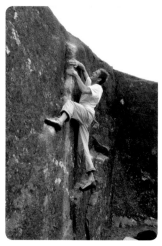

⬆ **RAC boulders in North Wales, so called because the parking is in a layby that used to have an emergency RAC phone box.**

⬆ **Noel Craine on Lordy, Lordy – his own problem in the Meadows, Llanberis, North Wales.**

There was a time when the hardest moves on boulders were leagues ahead of those possible on proper climbs, but now there's only a marginal difference, and some might suggest there's none at all. Though the focus of bouldering as a sport tends towards the harder and more technical end of climbing standards, it's important to know that easier and very worthwhile problems exist and, like climbing itself, you don't have to be an elite performer to have fun.

Two main grading systems are used for bouldering as follows:

▪ **Font** Named after Fontainebleau, near Paris, where there's an infinite number and variety of boulders, this system has grades from Font 3 to Font 8c, with sub-divisions of a, b, c and + once Font 6 is reached.

▪ **V-Scale** Developed by American climber John Sherman, initially for the huge bouldering region of Hueco Tanks in Texas, this system runs from V0 to V15.

It's incredibly difficult to make comparisons between bouldering grades and sport or trad grades for rock climbing, but for those who would like somewhere to begin V0 or Font 4 are very rough approximations to a British technical grade of 5a/5b. I hope that's vague enough…

⬇ **Talfarach at Porth Ysgo, a coastal destination on the Lleyn peninsula.**

⬇ **Steep Arête 6b+ is in a remote cwm – requiring a long walk! – on the flanks of Cnicht in North Wales; the rock is delightful rough dolerite.**

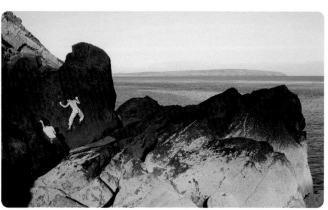

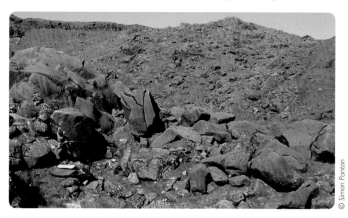

© Simon Panton

© Simon Panton

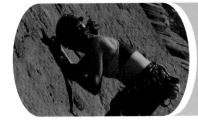

STYLES OF CLIMB

In time, and with more than a few climbs under your belt, it's likely that you'll develop a taste for certain styles of climb. There are many different styles that are largely differentiated by angle and the scarcity or otherwise of handholds and footholds.

Low-angle slabs of smooth rock with very few features are known as slab climbs. As the angle of the slab increases (to around 60 degrees or a little more) and the features diminish, the climbing becomes more difficult and, if lacking bolt protection, potentially quite dangerous as running belays may also diminish in number. Bold, steep and poorly protected slab climbing isn't for the faint-hearted, yet there are climbers who relish the very thought.

On rock walls from around 60 degrees through to vertical and further to the slightly overhanging angles, handholds need to be bigger to make the climb easier. A steep, overhanging wall of rock festooned with obliging handholds and footholds is generally known as 'thuggy' climbing, where strength and brawn are required – along with technique of course. Steep rock walls with small but positive holds are climbed with strong fingers and good technique, known as 'fingery' climbing. There are climbers who excel at these particular styles.

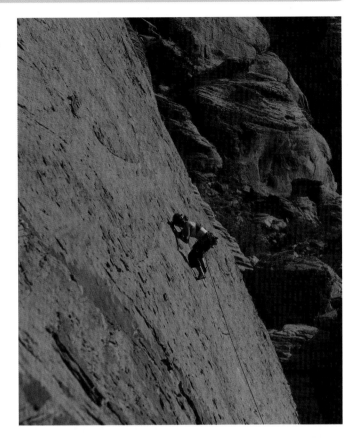

➔ **Bold, thin slab climbing at Red Rocks near Las Vegas. Bold because the protection is not only spaced a very long way apart but also because the bolts are very old and of doubtful solidity and thin because all the holds are very tiny, difficult to locate and not particularly reassuring. It's still an amazingly enjoyable and gratifying climb.**

ROCK FOR CLIMBING

Limestone, sandstone, gritstone, slate, granite, quartzite, dolerite, rhyolite and conglomerate are all rock types suited to climbing. In fact the only rock types that can't be climbed with hands and feet are chalk and mudstone.

Some rock types have unique features, such as the following:

- **LIMESTONE** has pockets, sharp flakes, smooth slabs and calcite flows known as 'tufas'; as limestone becomes polished very quickly with the passage of numerous feet and hands, popular climbs at limestone crags can feel very slippery and shiny.
- **SANDSTONE** is rough but relatively soft and easily eroded.
- **GRITSTONE** is quite coarse, very rough and not kind to skin; similar to sandstone, it features generally quite rounded handholds.
- **SLATE** is slippery, friable and sharp.

- **GRANITE** varies from fairly compact forms through to large grains, and can be exceptionally abrasive – so friction properties are excellent.
- **QUARTZITE** is a super-heated form of sandstone and offers a mix of characteristics.
- **DOLERITE** is like a halfway house between gritstone and sandstone, slightly more compact but with excellent friction properties.
- **RHYOLITE** offers a massive variety of styles of climbing and forms most of the mountain crags in England and Wales; it ranges from rough to fairly smooth, and contains many crack features.
- **CONGLOMERATE** looks like boulders and pebbles mixed together with hard-set mud. Despite looking a bit scary, it can be interesting to climb on because the embedded bits of rock can be of almost any type.

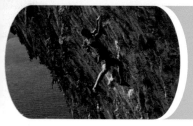

VISITING OTHER AREAS

To describe the infinite variety of rock climbing available around the world would require a lengthy tome running to several volumes, so this is only the briefest overview.

UK

Devotees of rock climbing in Britain have an almost unparalleled variety of climbing contained within a compact and accessible country that can claim to be the birthplace of rock climbing and the ethical epicentre of world climbing.

You can climb on sea cliffs, remote high mountain crags, roadside sport crags, disused quarries and accessible mountain crags. You can experience limestone, sandstone, gritstone, granite, slate, rhyolite, dolerite, quartzite and shale. You can climb routes from a few metres to several hundred metres long.

The main regions for rock climbing are North Wales, Pembrokeshire, the Peak District, the Yorkshire Dales, Glencoe,

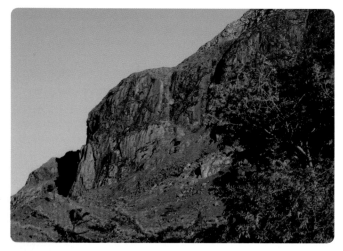

⬆ **Dinas Mot, Llanberis Pass.**

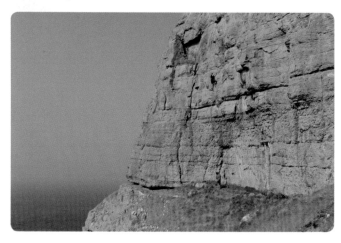

⬆ **Limestone sport climbing near Llandudno, North Wales.**

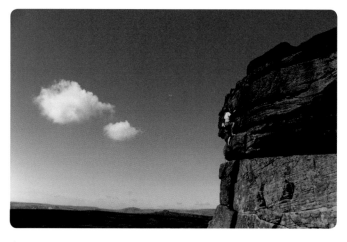

⬆ **Stanage Edge is a short bus ride from Sheffield.**

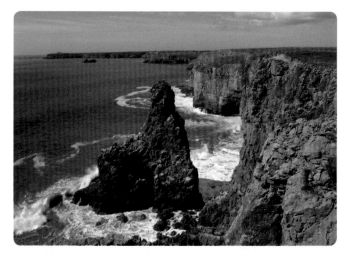

⬆ **The Pembrokeshire coastline attracts rock climbers from all over the world.**

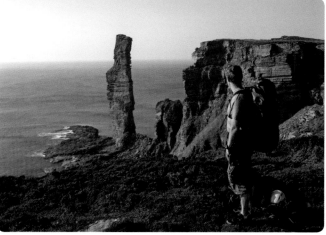

⬆ **The Old Man of Hoy, far in the north-west of the Orkney Islands, Scotland.**

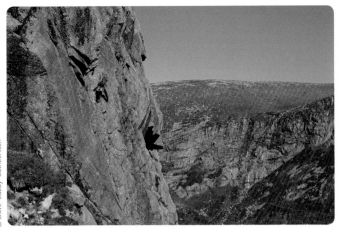

© Dave 'Cubby' Cuthbertson

⬆ **A climber on Mousetrap VS 4c Creag an Dubh Loch in the Cairngorm mountains in Scotland – a classic mountaineering climb with all the attributes of a true mountain setting that's both remote and inspirational.**

Ben Nevis, the north-western Highlands and the southern sandstone areas

EUROPE

Tens of thousands of rock climbs in diverse cultural environments make Europe the premier foreign destination for UK-based climbers.

In France alone you could spend a lifetime climbing. Sport climbing venues abound, some created with financial help from local communities and councils, and they cater for all standards, from the simplest to the hardest. In the south of France the Gorge du Verdon has climbs that take many hours to ascend, and the cliff of Céüse in the Haute Provence is where some of the worlds' hardest climbs can be found. Mountain routes that are several pitches long can be found in areas surrounding the higher peaks of the Alps.

In Switzerland perhaps the most famous venue is around the Grimsel and Furka passes. Huge granite slabs, with some routes of several pitches in length, provide interesting and sometimes scary climbing at an altitude that's cooling during summer months. Another significant crag is the multi-pitch venue of Rätikon, where long, bolted routes of mainly high-end difficulty abound.

The islands of Sardinia and Corsica offer an intensity of varied rock, largely gnarled and rough granite in Corsica, and perfect, pocketed, compact limestone in Sardinia. Sicily has long been a climbing destination for Italian climbers but is rapidly gaining popularity among foreign visitors.

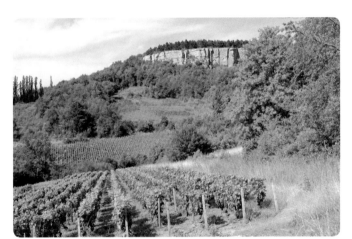

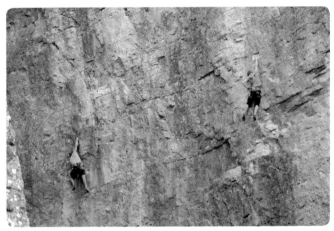

⬆ ⬈ **Burgundy, France, more famous for wine than for climbing, but like good wine...**

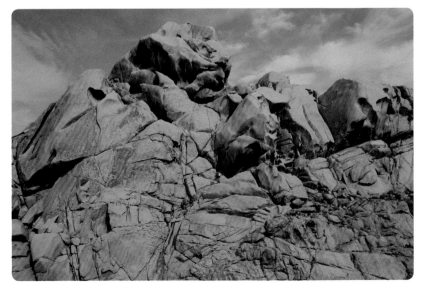

⬅ **Capo di Testa in northern Sardinia is a unique sculptured land of granite, perfect for rock climbers.**

➡ **Much of Sardinia is limestone, from steep tufa climbing to scary thin slabs – and everything in between.**

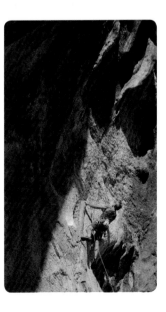

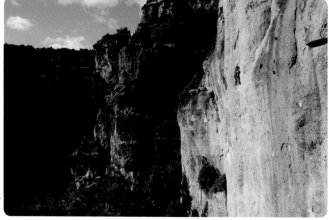

© Ray Wood

⬆ **Mandragora 7c in Siurana, which is on Spain's Costa Daurada, a few kilometres inland from the coast and a popular destination for 'winter sun' seeking climbers.**

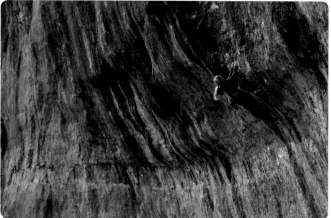

© Ray Wood

⬆ **Anabolica 8a at Siurana: this area has climbs of all grades but is noted for its quality climbs at the highest levels; there are a number of 'must do' climbs for those who aspire to hard sport climbing.**

The Costa Daurada in Spain is an amazing place to visit. Many British climbers head there during the long autumn and winter seeking sunshine and warmth, even in January, and out of season cheap flights and tourist accommodation make it particularly attractive.

Rewarding climbing can also be found in Croatia, Serbia, Slovenia and Greece. The tiny Greek island of Kalymnos is one of the most intensely developed climbing venues in Europe and has a justifiably good reputation for quality rock and climbing variety.

USA

From desert sandstone cracks and towers to the massive rock walls of Yosemite, and much more in between, the USA has everything to offer the rock climber of any standard. Whatever their aspirations in climbing, a visit to North America must surely be on everyone's wish-list. The only difficulty is choosing where to go!

The mecca for big wall climbing (multi-day climbs often requiring skills of a different nature to crag climbing) has to be Yosemite National Park. The Nose of El Capitan is probably the most famous long climb anywhere in the world and stands a monumental 900m (2,900ft) above the valley floor, dominating every vista in the valley. The original ascent of this magnificent feature took 45 days between July 1957 and

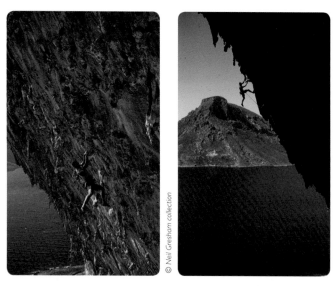

© Neil Gresham collection

⬆ **Kalymnos, Greece, is a climbing paradise where the island's inhabitants have welcomed climbers with open arms and provided equipment to make climbs.**

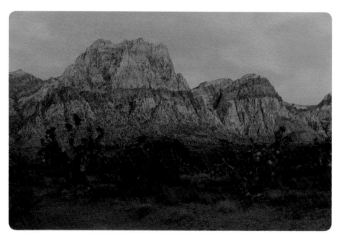

⬆ **Red Rocks, Nevada. Just beyond the city limits of Las Vegas lies one of the world's most outstanding climbing areas with over 1,700 rock climbs, sport and trad, from the easiest and shortest through to the hardest multi-day, multi-pitch challenges.**

➔ **The awesome Nose of El Capitan in the Yosemite National Park: this massive rock face towers 900m above the valley floor.**

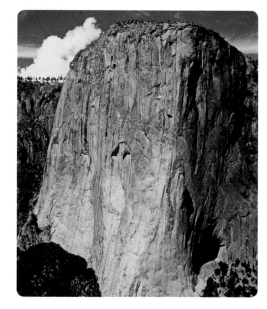

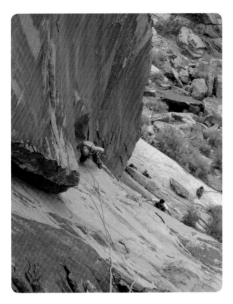

⬆ **The Great Red Book, Red Rocks: a classic, moderately graded climb, only two pitches long but a lasting memory.**

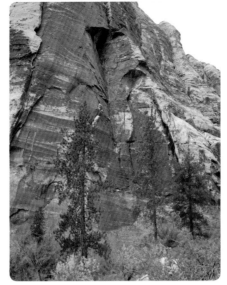

⬆ **Dark Shadows, Red Rocks: climbers can be seen in the corner feature.**

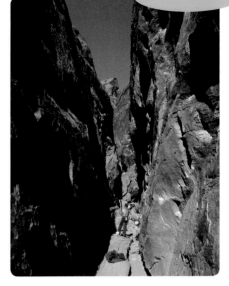

⬆ **Black Corridor, Red Rocks: a very popular sports climbing venue with easy access.**

November 1958, and even today many climbers attempting the ascent will spend two, three or even four days on the face. It has also been climbed without resorting to aid and, even more remarkably, it has been soloed, without ropes or gear of any kind! The first completely free ascent was by Lynn Hill in 1993 over four days, but a year later she returned to climb it free in just over 23 hours. Tommy Caldwell made the first sub-12-hour ascent in 2005, and in 2012 two climbers roped together and climbing simultaneously made the ascent in an extraordinary two hours, 23 minutes and 51 seconds.

Yosemite has many other faces equally well known to climbers, such as Middle Cathedral, Glacier Point Apron and the imposing Half Dome.

For shorter cragging-style climbs, venues abound, with highlights such as Smith Rocks (Oregon), the Shawangunks (New York State), and Tahquitz Rock and Suicide Rock (California). For a superb mixture of long multi-pitch climbs and single-pitch sport and trad routes, Red Rocks, on the outskirts of Las Vegas, is unbeatable.

AUSTRALIA

Deadly Snakes and spiders might conjure up images of outback Australia, but climbing venues can be found in abundance.

Mount Arapiles in Victoria, Mount Buffalo granite nearby and the Grampians close to Sydney all offer a variety of rock adventures on short sport climbs and long multi-pitch routes.

AFRICA

The world-famous Table Mountain at the southern tip of Africa is an unlikely place to find good rock climbing but it has one of the most spectacular mid-grade climbs anywhere in the world. In the South African grading system Jacob's Ladder is graded 16, which equates to about Very Severe in UK standards. The second pitch of this spectacular climb begins with an unlikely hand traverse followed by an incredibly steep, well-protected, 'juggy' arête. The belay stance at the end is one of the most awe-inspiring anywhere.

Elsewhere in the Cape region are the granite domes of Paarl Rocks, the sandstone of Elsie's Peak and, in the heart of the wine-growing region, Du Toits Peak.

Further north is the famous Rocklands, where multi-pitch and single-pitch sport climbing combine with outstanding bouldering. A must-do climb is Celestial Journey at Wolfberg Cracks.

Just outside Johannesburg is the region of Magaliesberg, a sandstone gorge offering interesting trad climbs, and a few hour's drive west is an area known as 'The Restaurant at the end of the Universe' – worth a visit just to say you've been there!

In Morocco the Todra Gorge and, more specifically, the mecca of Tafraoute provide a variety of single- and multi-pitch sport and longer trad climbs on near-perfect rock in a near-perfect setting.

AND ELSEWHERE...

If that isn't enough to satiate your appetite for rock climbing, you could climb in Norway, Jordan, Kyrgzstan, Thailand, Vietnam, Japan, New Zealand, Antarctica… wherever there's a rock to climb, someone will have climbed it.

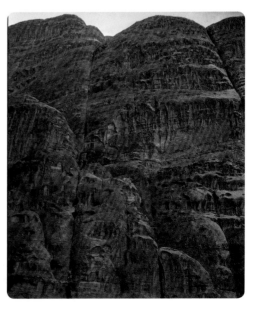

➡ **In the deserts of Jordan lies Wadi Rum, a vast area for the rock climber to explore and to savour the unusual nature of desert climbing.**

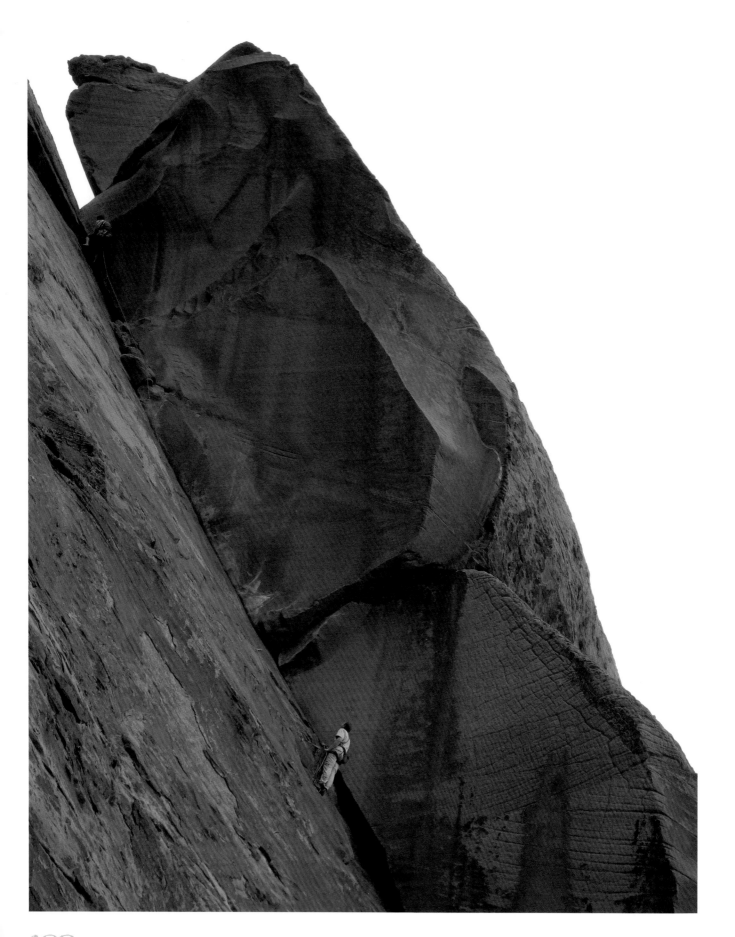

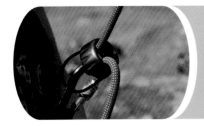

GLOSSARY

Abseil To descend on a rope using a friction device attached to the harness.

Aid To use a piece of protection equipment as an artificial handhold or foothold; there are climbs that are entirely 'aid'.

Air time Relates to the length of the leader fall taken; 'Big Air' normally means a very long fall.

Anchor To secure yourself to the rock face in order to belay a leader or a second; you can have single or multiple anchors.

Belay Method used to safeguard a climber while he or she is climbing.

Belay device Used to help safeguard a climber.

Belay/Abseil loop The sewn loop on a harness linking the waist belt and leg loops together.

Beta Prior knowledge of moves or specific information that prepares you for the climb.

Bolt A pre-placed piece of permanent protection.

Bomber Usually refers to a piece of protection as being sound or 'bombproof'.

Bottom roping Safeguarding a climber from the ground; the rope passes through a pulley-style anchor at the top of the climb.

Bouldering A low-level form of climbing and a sport in its own right.

Camming device Used for a running belay or an anchor in a crack in the rock.

Central loop Formed by the rope when you tie it in to the harness as per the manufacturer's recommendation.

Crux The most difficult part of a climb or pitch.

Dead rope The rope that doesn't go directly to the climber when he or she is being belayed; sometimes called the 'controlling rope'.

Decking out To hit the ground at the end of a fall – not recommended.

Desperate A really hard sequence of moves; can also be applied to a whole climb.

Disco leg An uncontrollable shaking of one (or even both) legs brought on by fear; sometimes known as 'sewing-machine leg'.

Dogging Failing to climb a route cleanly, without falling or resting on gear; usually done several times to help overcome a problem.

Exposed The feeling of being a very long way off the ground in an airy position; may lead to dry-mouth syndrome.

Flapper A small 'flap' of skin on the end of a fingertip caused by a pulling force over a small sharp hold; extremely painful and may stop you climbing.

Free climbing Climbing a route using only natural rock holds for hands and feet; climbers are normally roped together.

Gear loop The loops on a harness to which you can clip equipment.

Head-pointing Applied to trad routes where the climb is practised first on a rope from above and then led, possibly with some protection pre-placed.

Leader The climber who ascends the route first.

Live rope The rope that goes directly to the climber who's being belayed.

Lob To fall off.

Lower-off (noun) The fixed point at the top of a sport climb from which climbers are lowered back to the ground.

Lower off (verb) To lower a climber down after a climb.

Nuts Wedge-shaped or hexagonal nuts on wire, rope or tape that are wedged into cracks to make running belays or anchors; generically called 'rocks' and 'hexes'.

On sight To turn up at a climb with no prior knowledge of the intricacies of the route and ascend without resorting to artificial aid or falling.

Pay out To feed rope out through a belay device; normally for the leader but a second may ask for slack rope to be paid out.

Protection All the paraphernalia of crack protection and slings used to protect and safeguard the climb; often abbreviated to Pro or Gear.

Prusik A knot formed using a thin cord loop wrapped around the main climbing rope; such knots include the French Prusik used in abseil safety.

Pumped Tired arms that seem as if they may not hold you on to the rock for very much longer.

Red-point This is where the climber, usually on a sport route, will make a trial ascent, placing quickdraws and practising all moves (but very often falling and re-trying them several times). On reaching the top, the climber is lowered back to the ground and then leads the climb cleanly with no falls or rests, and with the quickdraws already in place.

Rest To take a break on a climb, usually at a place where you can take one or both hands off the rock.

Running belay Protection arranged by the leader using wedge-shaped nuts, hexagonal nuts, slings, camming devices or bolts; often shortened to 'runner'.

Sandbag A climb that belies its grade and is actually much harder than suggested. You can also 'sandbag' your mate by sending him or her on a climb that you know is much more difficult than the grade – usually one where you've already been sandbagged yourself!

Second The climber who follows the leader up the climb.

Sport climbing A style of climbing where the protection for the leader is permanently in place.

Stance A place part way up a climb or at the top where you secure yourselves while belaying each other.

Taking in A leader takes in the rope while the second climbs up.

Top roping A style of climbing where the climber is belayed from the top of the climb but walks around to the top to make the anchor and create the stance.

Trad climbing Derived from 'traditional climbing', this is the purest form of climbing, where all protection is placed by the climbers and then removed as they ascend; sometimes called 'adventure climbing'.

Thuggy climbing Steep climbing, usually with big holds – but it can be very strenuous.

Thrutch Where climbing technique has to be abandoned, usually in a crack or chimney, and any part of the body used to gain upward progress.

AMERICAN TERMINOLOGY

Biner Krab
Locking biner Screwgate krab
Girth hitch Larksfoot
Stemming Bridging
Finger lock Finger jam
Abseil Rappel
SLCD Camming device (Spring-Loaded Camming Device)
Water bend Ring bend or tape knot
Munter hitch Italian hitch
Inside corner/open book Corner
Outside corner Arête
Mantle Mantleshelf

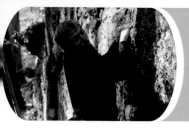

CLIMBING CALLS

THE KEY CALLS

Leader	Second	Definition
Safe!		Leader at top of climb or pitch and secured to anchors; second takes rope out of belay device.
	OK!	Has taken rope out of belay device.
Taking in!		Hauls up the slack rope between two climbers hand over hand and stacks neatly on belay stance.
	That's me!	Rope has come tight.
Climb when ready!		Leader has put rope in belay device and checked all is safe and sound; second can untie from anchor points.
	Climbing!	Second untied from anchors and ready to move; leader can now anticipate having to hold a falling second.
OK!		Acknowledges readiness.

OTHER CALLS

Leader	Second	Definition
	Go for it!	Or similar… Encouragement to a leader to help him climb the pitch when showing signs of faltering.
Watch me here!		Leader feeling nervous or very concerned, and needs reassurance as above.
	Hang on a mo!	Or similar… Second has a tangle in the rope and needs to sort it out.
Take me!		Leader will fall or thinks he may fall.
	I've got you!	Reassurance to leader, but needs to be prepared to pay out rope if leader suddenly decides to make moves upwards.
Slack!		Second not paying out enough rope for leader; or panic clip of runner; or leader has too much rope drag for rope to run.
	Take in!	Second has too much slack rope; or call is a precursor to a fall if the rope is already as tight as it could be.
That's a bomber!		Leader has found a really good runner placement and everyone can relax.
Expletives…	Expletives…	Usually spells trouble ahead…
Whoops of joy…	Whoops of joy…	All is good with the world, the climb or pitch has been conquered – and everyone is happy.

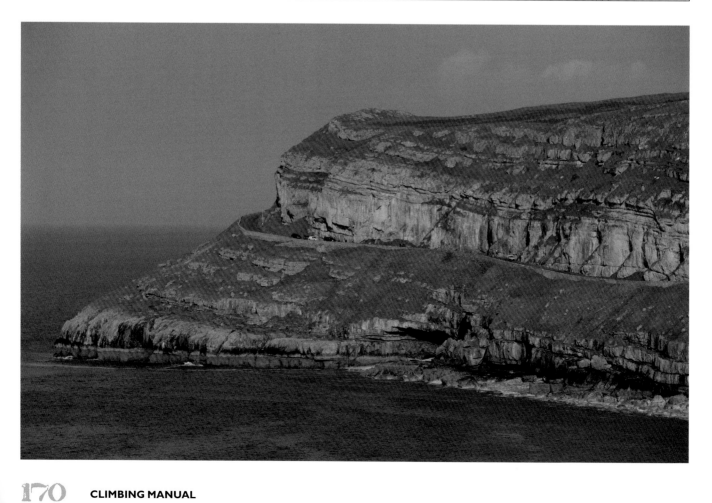

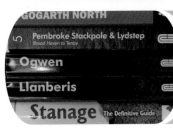

RESOURCES

Listed here are a small selection of resources on the internet that you may find helpful.

COURSES AND INSTRUCTION

www.bmg.org.uk British Mountain Guides is the national association that provides a whole variety of opportunities for instructional courses and private guiding and tuition. Members of the association have to go through a long, arduous process of training and assessment in all mountain sport disciplines as well as gaining considerable experience to a high standard of performance. This makes them the highest qualified of all outdoor professionals, able to work anywhere in the world.

www.ami.org.uk The Association of Mountaineering Instructors is also a UK-based organisation. Linked to Mountain Training (MT), the co-ordinating body for all mountain training schemes in the UK, they train and assess individuals to teach rock climbing among other mountaineering disciplines.

Mountain Training introduced a new coaching award system in late 2013. There are three award levels: Foundation, Development and Performance Coach. Each level brings together three important strands of a coach's personal and supervisory experience of climbing: a technical understanding of What to Coach; the Safe Supervision of activity and a greater knowledge of How to Coach more effectively.

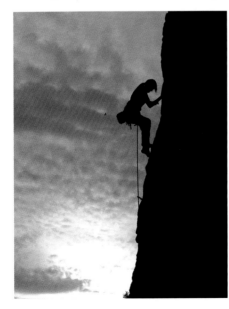

These are the two main professional qualifications. Others are the Single-Pitch Award (SPA) and the Climbing Wall Award (CWA), which are basic qualifications of competence to look after beginners in an introductory manner on outdoor single-pitch venues and indoor climbing walls.

www.masterclasscoachingacademy.com Rock climbing coaching courses are run in the UK at indoor climbing walls and abroad at selected climbing destinations. One-to-one or group coaching classes will help you develop skills and techniques to enable you climb better and harder. Courses are focussed mainly on sport climbing and bouldering. Masterclass Climbing Coaches have the highest level of climbing coach qualification achievable in the UK. Coaches climb to the highest standards and are able to offer advice on training programmes as well as personal performance.

General resources

www.ukclimbing.com A great website for UK climbing in particular, but also a valuable resource for worldwide information.

www.thebmc.co.uk The British Mountaineering Council (BMC) is the national body for mountaineering sport in the UK. It offers travel insurance specific to climbing as well as a host of other advice on all safety aspects. It is also responsible for negotiating and ensuring continued access to crags and cliffs around the UK.

www.mcofs.org.uk The Mountaineering Council of Scotland (MCofS) is the organisation with similar responsibilities in Scotland to those of the BMC.

www.rockfax.com A publisher that offers an excellent range of UK guidebooks as well as other titles for popular areas in Europe and beyond.

www.groundupclimbing.com A publisher based in North Wales with a small catalogue of first-rate guidebooks including the fantastic *North Wales Bouldering Guide*.

www.climbers-club.co.uk Publisher of definitive climbing guides to Wales, south-west and southern England.

www.frcc.co.uk The Fell and Rock Climbing Club – publisher of definitive guides to the Lake District.

www.smc.org.uk Scottish Mountaineering Council – publisher of definitive guides to Scotland's climbing.

MAGAZINES

www.climber.co.uk and **www. climbmagazine.com** Fascinating magazines that inspire you to travel to destinations and also have lots of information on techniques and skills.

CLIMBING EQUIPMENT MANUFACTURERS

The key equipment manufacturers are listed here. Their websites don't simply offer a catalogue of equipment available but they also have fascinating articles on equipment use, testing, up-to-date safety considerations and pages about the exploits of their sponsored athletes – they're all truly inspiring with outstanding photography.

www.dmmclimbing.com
www.edelrid.de
www.arcteryx.com
www.wildcountry.co.uk
www.blackdiamondequipment.com
www.petzl.com
www.lasportiva.com
www.fiveten.com
www.scarpa.co.uk

NON-UK RESOURCES

www.climbing.com The website of US magazine *Climbing*; inspiring articles, reviews of latest equipment, destinations.

www.rockclimbing.com All manner of information about climbing around the world but particularly useful if you're visiting the USA.

www.supertopo.com An essential resource for the USA particularly with up-to-date information on climbing areas; Publisher of Guidebooks and topos.

www.climbing.com.au Comprehensive information about climbing in Australia.

www.thecrag.com Database of crags and climbs in OZ and around the world.

www.climb.co.za Everything you need for climbing in South Africa.

www.climb.co.nz New Zealand.

www.cosiroc.org France.

www.planetmountain.com Italy.

www.escuelasdeescalada.com Spain.

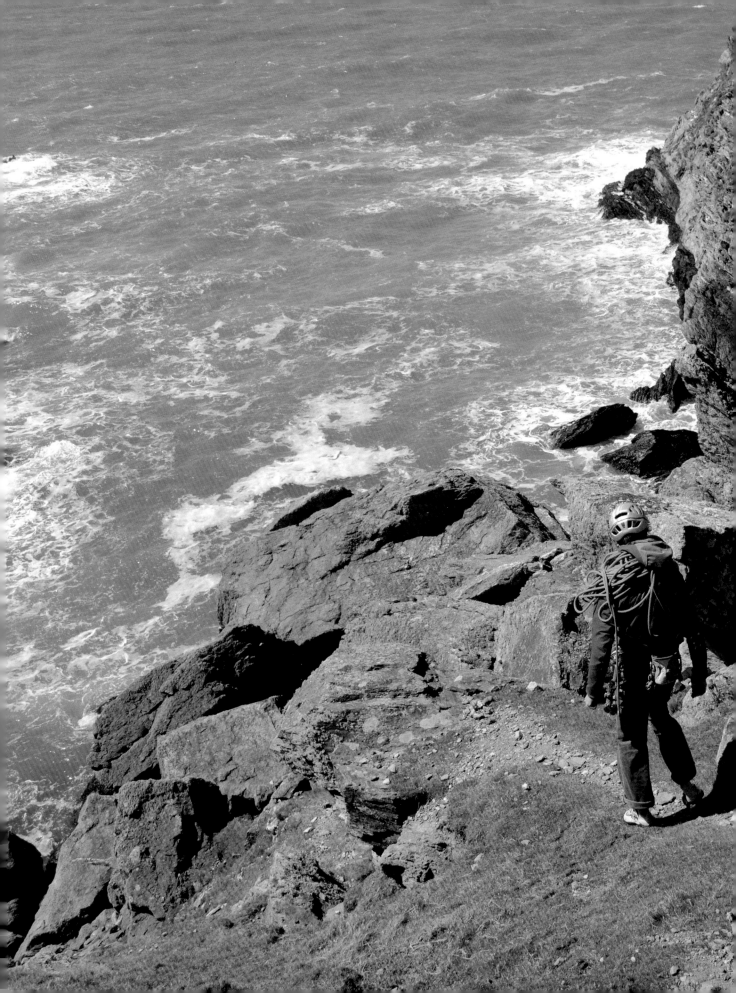